Gone Viral

GONE VIRAL

How Covid Drove the
World Insane

JUSTIN HART

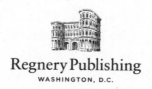

Regnery Publishing
WASHINGTON, D.C.

Regnery® is a registered trademark and its colophon is a trademark of Salem Communications Holding Corporation

Cataloging-in-Publication data on file with the Library of Congress

ISBN: 978-1-68451-351-2
eISBN: 978-1-68451-370-3

Published in the United States by
Regnery Publishing,
A Division of Salem Media Group
Washington, D.C.
www.Regnery.com

Manufactured in the United States of America

10 9 8 7 6 5 4 3 2 1

Books are available in quantity for promotional or premium use. For information on discounts and terms, please visit our website: www.Regnery.com.

To Jenny,

For standing with me on the pillars of life.

To Mom and Dad,

For the heritage, love, family, and faith that will live on for eternity.

CONTENTS

Debunking the Myths of Covid

'm not a health care expert. Normally I wouldn't insert myself into someone else's domain, but the powers that be seemed to have *no* problem inserting themselves into mine: they closed in on my business, my church, my kids' education, my health, my grocery store, my gym, my coffee shop, my barber—you name it, and some government entity was there with strangling regulations or an order to shut the thing down entirely.

My business was simply killed outright. I'm an executive consultant for a host of various industries in my day job. I help companies, nonprofits, and political campaigns visualize the way they're performing through interactive dashboards, kick-butt charts, and the like. Plus, at the beginning of the pandemic, most of my income came from running companies that offered exclusive golf excursions for baby boomers, one-on-one consulting for college-bound kids, and a high-end vacation club for wealthy families. The pandemic killed that side of my business dead as a doornail. Within weeks of the pandemic hitting, I had no clients to speak of.

I'm not one to sit around, so I threw myself into the thing that everyone was talking about—coronavirus. With my good friend and colleague Aaron Ginn, I formed a rag-tag bunch of analysts, chart-makers, and lay activists who were ready to be rid of our health over-lords and get our lives back to normal. We called our group *Rational Ground*.

Eventually, Rational Ground started publishing on a daily basis with our Substack (covidreason.substack.com), our website (RationalGround.com), and our primary social media presence on Twitter. We would come to be one of the leading voices of reason in the fight against insane Covid policies.

Since the failure of PCR testing, we discussed the age-stratified risk of Covid and the death-certificate details on COVID-19 deaths. We made interactive charts that helped users visualize what the data actually *meant* in their lives. We brought up the sheer lunacy of the stay-at-home orders and pointed out the true low, low risk of the virus and its effects for children.

It was quality material people weren't finding anywhere else, and we gained followers at a rapid rate. By fall 2020 one of those followers was Dr. Scott Atlas, who at the time was a key advisor to the Trump administration on its COVID-19 response. In fact, Atlas even asked us to produce charts for him, a project we gladly undertook. These charts were televised nationally and used as evidence against the one-size-fits-all approach that had characterized the White House response up until Dr. Atlas's arrival.

But, like Sauron's eye scanning Middle Earth for the Ring of Power, the powers that be were on the lookout for any who would question their authority. The attention we received caught their atten-tion, and they were *not* amused. In the summer of 2021, my accounts on Twitter and Facebook were suspended for publishing some of the data that our Rational Ground colleagues produced. Indeed, many of our colleagues would have social media accounts suspended or altogether taken down over the course of the pandemic.

Our particular offense was posting an infographic produced by one of our pseudonymous Twitter friends entitled: "Masking Children is Impractical and Not Backed by Research or Real World Data." In twelve squares on the graphic, we presented the facts. These notions were simply common-sense deductions based on evidence that many folks can agree upon. Each point was rigorously backed up with peer-reviewed or pre-print studies. Nothing was out-there or fringe about these ideas. The information included the facts that children are at very low risk from COVID-19, that teachers do not face an increased risk from children—a simple reality that the teachers' unions have made verboten—along with the obvious points that the effectiveness of masks is not conclusive, that masking children is unrealistic, and that improper masking is common and unsanitary and can cause a variety of health issues. Maybe the most telling point was that masks can hinder speech development in children and the effect on deaf and disabled kids is particularly devastating.[1]

As with all things Twitter in those days, it was unclear why it and other social media platforms suspended our accounts for benign and well-supported posts like these. They never gave specifics but pointed to vague user agreements. But we all knew the why of it in the larger sense—and where the real instigation to wipe us from the internet came from—although some were reluctant to admit it at first. The banning impulse came from the very top.

In July 2021, White House press secretary Jen Psaki said, "We've increased disinformation research and tracking within the Surgeon General's office. We're flagging problematic posts for Facebook that spread disinformation." Psaki also revealed that the White House effort to suppress free speech reaches all the way to the level of senior staff for President Biden.[2] Although we didn't know about it at the time, plans were even underway to establish a "Ministry of Truth" in the Department of Homeland Security known as the Disinformation Governance Board, where it would have a dedicated law enforcement wing to back up its edicts. Pressuring social media platforms to kick people like us off was merely the tip of the new censorship spear the government was honing.

Did these suspensions and tactics scare us? Not a whit. Maybe we were naïve. Maybe we were a bunch of data nerds in over our heads. But we were people for whom the truth mattered. We were the types who loved sifting that truth out of a mound of data. Most of all we wanted to regain our lives—and the lives of our friends and families.

My wife Jenny and I have a Brady Bunch–like situation. We have eight kids between us. The three youngest are ours. Jenny has two daughters, eighteen and fourteen, and I have three older kids. So, at any given moment, at least four kids are usually traipsing about the halls getting ready for school. All of that changed after Thanksgiving 2021. Our fourteen-year-old's private school sent us a note that she would have to quarantine at home for the rest of 2021. Why? Was she even sick?

It turned out to have nothing to do with her. Because someone in the school musical had tested positive for Covid, and because our daughter is unvaccinated, she had no recourse—she would be forced to miss the rest of school in December including the Christmas concert. Her friends who were vaccinated could go on their merry way and back to school. Furthermore, the student who contracted Covid was vaccinated himself. School policy prohibited the test-to-stay option because the students weren't masked at the play practice. No one was sick besides the fully vaccinated student who had tested positive for Covid. Our daughter had been singled out for exclusion because she was not vaccinated.

Of course, she was devastated.

I was livid—and I still am. This is a private school here in San Diego and the only high school to remain open the entire 2020–21 school season. Jenny had sent her daughters there for years. Was there loyalty from the school to Jenny and the commitment and tuition she'd poured into the school for over a decade? Not a whit. We had to conclude that the school's mission lacks courage as a component and is not aligned with our values. I had to fight with the school to keep my daughter in classes.

Meanwhile, the state licensing board came down hard on our kids' preschool in late 2021. The director of this preschool (which has been operating for thirty-eight years) was determined to fight to keep masks off of our kids. She knows the learning harm they cause the very young. Try teaching a four-year-old how to pronounce the letter *H* through a mask!

The California state licensing folks made a surprise visit to the school, where they questioned *the kids*, asking aloud why so many of them weren't wearing a mask. My five-year-old replied: "Because my dad filled out a form, and I don't have to, and he doesn't believe in them!"

Soon after, they threatened to shut down the school.

Now those kids must acquire a medical note attached to their file to avoid masking. When we went to the pediatrician to ask for it, she replied that she believed masks work. Well, I think they don't work for five-year-old kids. My daughter's happiness and development now depend on me—her father—being able to obtain a note from someone outside our family to exempt her from the practice. The government of California has forced me into a fight with my pediatrician when the two of us should be allies in promoting my daughter's health and well-being.

I am part of three generations here in California. Jenny's California roots go back to the 1800s. This would be a hard place to leave. But we do not want to live a life subject to the whims of unelected bureaucrats. When I pressed the leadership of the school, they pointed me to a letter from San Diego County supervisor Nathan Fletcher, who in no uncertain terms threatened all schools, public or private, with serious consequences if they did not adhere to the mandates. In the end, our private school rolled over meekly. It lacked the will to fight for the education of the children it claimed to serve.

In just one of numerous examples, the lunch attendant and school nurse told the eighth-grade class that they should sit perpendicular to the lunch bench and not face their other classmates. Presumably Covid only transmits in one direction. It's this kind of madness that gives us pause to realize that the virus of the mind is far more damaging than the virus itself.

Many of those who joined Rational Ground and what we came to call Team Reality had similar experiences. Life isn't always fair, and we adults are willing to bear with the challenges foisted on us, but when the government's insane rules harm our children, watch out.

PART 1

THE MOTHER OF ALL COVID MYTHS

CHAPTER 1

Interventions Have No Costs! WRONG.

The butterfly effect is a component of chaos theory noting the potential for small changes to greatly impact a complex system. To wit, a butterfly flaps his wings, and a chain of events conspires to cause a hurricane on the other side of the world. While this is an academically debated notion, its general application to the pandemic will be studied for ages. Consider perhaps the greatest undergirding myth of the pandemic: asymptomatic spread.

The dreads of asymptomatic transmission (infecting someone else when you don't know you are infected to begin with) has caused more damage to American health than the virus ever could. Early in the pandemic, National Institute of Allergy and Infectious Disease director Dr. Anthony Fauci took to the microphone and very frankly stated that "asymptomatic transmission has never been the driver of outbreaks."[1]

Yet within weeks this assumption was thrown out the window by Fauci himself and the leadership of what we came to call "Team Apocalypse." That one decision was the triggering moment for masks, quarantines, business closures, stay-at-home orders, and hospital madness.

Mask Wearing Is Unscientific Nonsense

Consider masks. Masking the public was based on the premise that anyone could be a super spreader. Symptomless Covid was thought to be just as deadly and transmissible as the real thing. Masking was considered an intervention if you were sick, but now it became a better-safe-than-sorry mandate as everyone was masked, because, well, you never know. It would be over a year before the CDC (Centers for Disease Control and Prevention) admitted that aerosolized transmission was probably the main driver of Covid. The spread was *not* due to asymptomatic people. Let that sink in. The virus spread because it was everywhere around you if you *had* symptoms. The assumption that only droplets and spittle could contaminate another person wreaked havoc when combined with asymptomatic fears.

OSHA experts must have been red-faced when they realized what was being asserted about personal protection equipment (PPE). When cloth masks were widely dismissed as "facial decorations" the higher-quality N95 masks came out in force. Unlike cloth and surgical masks, these were intended to protect the wearer. Experts must have winced watching parents work these devices onto their children's faces considering there is *no* child certification for any N95 mask. According to OHSA (Occupational Safety and Health Administration) and the FDA (Food and Drug Administration), you're supposed to be clean-shaven when you wear one, too.

In this scenario, there was no cost analysis done. No psychologist was consulted. No fluid physicist was brought in. No education specialists. Their concerns were ever and always about stopping the virus at any cost. We gave the keys of the kingdom to people who hadn't seen a patient in thirty years. These were politicians, not actively working doctors. They certainly were not policy experts. They were entrenched bureaucrats.

Government Bureaucrats Are Terrible at Predicting the Future

Government is terrible at picking winners and losers and even worse at predicting negative outcomes. Take the state government of California. In 2008 the legislature in Sacramento passed a bill essentially outlawing Thomas Edison's most famous invention, the incandescent light bulb. They mandated instead the use of compact fluorescent lamps (CFL) as the go-to device to light everything. One lone conservative, Assemblyman Chuck DeVore, warned at the time that CFL light bulbs have some pretty toxic chemicals in them like neon and would need proper disposal. His colleagues dismissed his objections. One year later they were forced to allocate millions of dollars for proper disposal of the curlicue bulbs. In truth these bulbs were very inefficient, with high failure rates and an altogether undesirable lighting experience. Those of you who tried them might well recall the slight delay when you turned one on. What's more, this decision delayed the very efficient upcoming technology for light-emitting diode (LED) technology. It's likely that this one decision delayed the adoption of LEDs by a decade and artificially kept the price high while CFL usage peaked and then waned.

If the government had stayed out of the light-bulb business, the environmental benefits would have arrived years earlier than they did, at a fraction of the cost, and the light bulb itself casting an improved and more enjoyable light.

The pandemic saw its own share of stupid decisions made without weighing the costs and benefits of mandates or implementations. One of our most viral tweets during the pandemic showed a large turtle inhaling a mask with other turtles looking aghast as they floated in a sea of wet surgical face diapers (as we sometimes called them). As one report noted in 2021: "Most of these masks contain plastics or other derivatives of plastics. Therefore, this extensive usage of face masks generates [a] million tons of plastic wastes to the environments in a short span of time."[2]

Literally billions upon billions of masks have been produced over the course of the pandemic. The by-products of the *production* of the masks are enormous. The magnitude of discarded masks and PPE is even larger. One analyst noted that this was a "ecological disaster in the making."[3] No consideration was given to the recycling or disposal of these masks at the outset. Little has been done since then to mitigate the problems.

Lockdowns Are Ineffective and Destroy Lives

Lockdowns are the perhaps the best example of complete lack of forethought given to the impacts on the economy and on families across the world. Consider that massive waves of diseases in third-world countries continue to rise: an estimated 1.4 million additional tuberculosis deaths due to supply chain disruptions; 500,000 additional deaths related to HIV; and malaria deaths could double to 770,000 total per year.[4] It turns out the world is deeply connected. When you shut down the first-world economy, third-world problems explode.

As far as we know, there was no economic-impact analysis done. The massive grant, stimulus, and business-loan programs were slapped together to stem the bleeding as unemployment neared 14 percent across the country. As I note elsewhere, for every 1 percent uptick in unemployment, you can predict tens of thousands of deaths through loss of income, healthcare, substance abuse and other life-crushing impacts.[5]

What's more, did you ever hear a single member of the Covid-lockdown team, or any elected official, apologize for the impact this would have? It was just assumed that it was the thing to do, the only way forward. No input was asked from our representatives in Congress. Emergency powers granted to the executive branch were all that was needed. The only sympathetic note I could uncover was President Trump's repeated acknowledgement that the suffering that businesses endured was through "no fault of their own."[6]

Social Distancing Was and Is a Complete Joke

Consider the restaurant table and the changes you've witnessed from the pandemic. The tried-and-true ways of doing things might never come back. If you were allowed into the restaurant, there were limitations on the capacity under which the restaurant could operate. Even before those mandates took effect, social distancing requirements removed a swath of tables almost overnight. Seating was limited, and occasionally you were required to limit your fellow table guests to people you lived with. You wore a mask to the table as you entered the door. At some point at restaurants in some large cities like New York, Washington, D.C., and Los Angeles, you were required to show a vaccination card before entry. If you happened to have an unvaccinated child in your party, you were turned away.

As you approached the table, you noticed some changes. There was nothing on the table. CDC recommendations stated that no table should be preset with silverware and there should be no waters prefilled waiting for you. Salt and pepper shakers (long since gone in California) were now absent across most of the country. Instead of a physical menu, the ubiquitous QR code was used to pull up a menu on your tiny phone screen, assuming you had a phone and knew how to use this method. If menus were handed out, they had to be immediately disposed of.

Now that restaurants are reopened, the service is often abysmal. The lack of staff provides a terrible experience, from the dive diner to the five-star hotel. At one point I drove by to pick up some fast food for the family. A sign on the speaker near the menu noted: "We have no staff. We are closed." It was seven at night. One-third of all restaurants in California closed down permanently during the pandemic.

How many of those interventions are still in place? Have all of these "clean" interventions made you more or less confident about going out to dinner? How long will it take people to feel *normal* in these settings? Truth be told, when masks were removed in the summer of 2021 (before they were forced back on us), I felt a bit naked going into the grocery store without one.

Madness Claimed Society

Placating the neurosis which enveloped almost every American, the service industry bent over backwards to meet the growing fear of Covid everywhere. One Chick-fil-A drive-through placed their famously efficient order takers inside portable yellow bubble suits, fully masked. For many parts of the country dine-in would not return for over a year. To this day, almost all fast-food playgrounds are still closed for sanitary reasons. I'm told corporate lawyers are thrilled at this development given the general liability of Junior hurting himself on the McDonald's PlayPlace. So as not to offend even the most extreme sensibilities, Kentucky Fried Chicken placed their brand-defining catchphrase "finger-licking good" on sabbatical. Colonel Sanders handing out sanitary wipes just doesn't have a marketing ring to it. Cleanliness first, of course!

In sports arenas more nonsense ensued. In September 2020, the Washington Nationals general manager was ejected from the game for not wearing a mask—while sitting in the owner's suite, by himself.[7] In October, Dodgers third baseman Justin Turner was pulled from the game because he tested positive for coronavirus during the game.[8] Testing regimes mandated at the county and state levels got out of control. Dr. Allen Sills, chief medical officer for the NFL, took matters into his own hands and reduced the cycle threshold levels of the testing regime for NFL players so games could take place at all.[9]

Foreign governments tried all kinds of theater to demonstrate a combative effort against the virus. Taking their cue from China, numerous airlines across the globe were shown spraying down passengers as they arrived with some sort of mist. It's unclear what was intended, and perhaps it was just a placebo, an actual mist of water. In schools, malls, apartments, and stores, temperature takers and checkpoints became commonplace.

Social Control Has Become an End in Itself

Stay-at-home orders were seen as the measure of last resort according to all the literature, but across the globe the yo-yo effect of locking down and opening up was used quite frequently. You could sense the frustration in leaders as they tried to stem the tide of the variants. British prime minister Boris Johnson implemented another post-Christmas shelter-in-place order: "Now is the time to take action, because there is no alternative."[10] Leaders honestly could not stomach cases going up, so they pulled all the stops—to no avail.

Here in the United States, a slew of mobile apps sprouted up to facilitate the new swath of Covid regulations washing across every school district. "Mr. Owl" promised a quick and easy means for parents to check in their children on the way to school by affirming that they had no symptoms nor did anyone else in the household. If you failed to submit your record for that day, you promptly received a reminder call.

States and counties rolled out their own set of applications while major software firms developed tracking tools to help sniff out exposure points. In 2020 Apple introduced a Bluetooth-enabled feature on their popular iPhone. If you logged a positive case, it would inform people that you were around that they had been exposed to you.[11] Like a scene from *Invasion of the Body Snatchers*, if you were found ill—or worse, unvaccinated—the pointing digital finger was coming for you soon.

Governments Label Their Citizens as Killers

Before vaccines became a staple of all interventions, restaurants were required to log your name and number in case another patron called in with a positive case. Large school systems would dedicate fulltime resources to contact trace students who came down with COVID-19. In many places, county contact tracers would call folks who were registered with a positive test. A series of questions would follow and could become an accusatory interrogation in tone.

On county-data dashboards, charts were designed to convey the places where transmission occurred, but the results were, to say the least, unscientific, little better than guesswork.[12] According to contact tracers I spoke with, most of the people they reached (if they reached them at all) indicated that home transmission was the most common location followed by work exposure. The other percentages are simply based on asking this question: "Where have you gone over the past two weeks?"

Los Angeles County provided some of the most detailed data from their massive army of contact tracers in the most populated county in the country. They separated exposure by employee and patron. By the end of November 2020, the dashboard did not show a single transmission for a nonemployee.[13] Is it possible that California forced the closure of a third of all restaurants for no data-supported reason? It is indeed.

Disruptions were everywhere.

My wife and I ordered a new kitchen table in July of 2021. It did not arrive until March 2022. The delays were caused by numerous problems. The overseas manufacturer in Vietnam had closed its doors due to Covid outbreaks. When it finally made it across the sea by boat it was stuck in port for weeks. Why were the ports in California so backed up? The main reason: staffing and training. It was thought too dangerous for new crane operators to sit side-by-side with existing employees to learn the operations of these massive machines. Instead, they conducted virtual training with mediocre results leading to massive staff shortages at the ports. Every industry was impacted by these back-ups—and all because someone assumed that even though you weren't sick, you might be a killer.

PART 2

JUNK SCIENCE

CHAPTER 2

You Must Trust "The Science™"! WRONG.

Thanksgiving weekend came and went in 2021. The soothsayers of Team Apocalypse were wrong again—the sky didn't fall. Whole populations of families who dared to get together to celebrate were not wiped out. But that didn't stop NAID director Dr. Anthony Fauci. The Covid fatality rate doesn't hold a candle to the risk of standing between Dr. Fauci and a camera. After a few softball questions, the television host of CBS's *Face the Nation* asked Dr. Fauci about recent criticism of him from various corners. He replied:

> So, it's easy to criticize, but they're really criticizing science because I represent science. That's dangerous. To me, that's more dangerous than the slings and the arrows that get thrown at me. I'm not going to be around here forever, but science is going to be here forever. And if you damage science, you are doing something very detrimental to society long after I leave. And that's what I worry about.[1]

It is indeed dangerous to claim to represent science. Science doesn't need sales reps, since it is the conceptualization of physical reality itself as determined by experiment and data. What Fauci truly represented is the authoritarian State with a capital *S*.

Emails released through the Freedom of Information Act show Fauci to be a manipulative man of politics, deftly brushing off lengthy diatribes against him or mustering forces to push back on Team Reality. It really is quite the position to be in as the highest-paid federal employee in history to call upon the systematic enterprise of knowledge known as "science" to shield you from criticism.[2]

The damage wrought upon our science as an actual institution is incalculable. As Dr. Jay Bhattacharya noted, "The current generation of top public health leaders will need to step down before trust is restored."[3]

The science is *not* what they say it is, and you are not required to acquiesce to anyone's determinations but your own. Indeed, when someone declares himself to be the voice of authority in all things—run.

Science and the Application of Science Are Not the Same Thing

One keen realization our society must grapple with is that the science is separate from the application of that science. The science may indeed dictate that we experienced the spread of a highly transmissible, deadly, aerosolized viral respiratory pathogen, but it does not follow that you need to lose your job after that. Or that we ought to destroy the economy of a country. Or deprive a generation of children of proper learning.

Dr. Scott Atlas was lambasted by Team Apocalypse again and again for *not* being a virologist, but he was not sent to the White

House to fix "the science"—he was there to fix the policy. Indeed, Dr. Atlas had keen and deep expertise in the application of science to public policy, something Dr. Fauci has failed at again and again in his career.

Our Constitution affords U.S. citizens many enumerated rights and protections in our pursuit of happiness. Many of these endowed freedoms are couched in language specifically protecting us from the government writ large. While courts might attest to some extreme event placing some of these rights into dormancy, it did not give Dr. Fauci the right to put our rights, indeed our whole Constitution, into a coma.

The Institutions Lie. And Lie. And Lie.

Myriad once-trusted institutions have suffered greatly under the boom that Dr. Fauci and company lowered onto the American people and, frankly, the world.

The CDC has lost immense trust on all sides. From Dr. Robert Redfield's declaration that masks are better than vaccines to Dr. Rochelle Walensky selling you a non-sterilizing, *sterilizing* vaccine— this institution has wreaked the greatest havoc over the entire pandemic.[4] They manipulated data, hid data, ignored data, invented data, deleted data, dismissed data, and all around succumbed to political pressure. Whether it was from teachers' unions or a meddling White House, the CDC failed to provide any real leadership. With a budget of billions and over twenty thousand employees, the amount of work the CDC produced was puny and questionable at every step.

The National Institutes of Health (NIH) is another behemoth that needs a thorough cleaning. The NIH's (now) former director, Francis Collins, penned the infamous email calling out the signers of the Great Barrington Declaration.

"This proposal from the three fringe epidemiologists...seems to be getting a lot of attention—and even a co-signature from Nobel Prize winner Mike Leavitt at Stanford.... There needs to be a quick and devastating published take down of its premises."

Collins ends the email: "Is it underway?"[5]

If it wasn't, the establishment institutional heads got in gear and made sure to jumpstart the process of attempting to destroy the reputations of the signers, all manifestly qualified and fantastically credentialled scientists and doctors.

The National Institute of Allergy and Infectious Diseases (NIAID) headed by Dr. Fauci is one of the key culprits stalling any real progress on trust and communication around these vital topics. Fauci and Collins were keenly involved with all areas of research in this federal healthcare monstrosity and influenced millions of dollars in grants given every year. No wonder the spectrum of literature produced here did little to further any alternate views on lockdowns, masking, vaccines, and other COVID-19 implementations. The folks setting the policy also hold the purse strings.

It was obvious from the get-go that the structure of our county-centric administration of health policy was going to be problematic. These local health directors and advisors have little if any accountability. They are unelected bureaucrats and were given immense powers over the lives of citizens in their areas. The replete inconsistency with how federal health policy and information was conveyed to the public is an embarrassment. These county entities were given massive outlays of taxpayer dollars for the fruitless effort of contact tracing. The impact was not just on our wallets. As Jay Bhattacharya noted: "Hospital staffing shortages are at least in part due to rigidly enforced vaccine mandates and to mass asymptomatic testing and contact tracing. How many more people must suffer because of the monomaniacal focus on COVID at the expense of public health?"[6]

Contact tracing at the county level became a de facto quarantine machine, especially for students.

Most did it, many of us knowing it was pointless. But the pointlessness became the point. Comply, or you are bad person. Comply, or it's no more school for you.

And comply many people did, thinking they would weather the madness, counting the cost on their hearts and spirits as worth the sacrifice for their children's education. One more stricture, and the schools will open. Follow one more edict, and the playground tape will come off. And so it went for two plus years. So it *still* goes in many places. We were duped, but we also duped ourselves.

Public Trust Was Destroyed

The impact on the public trust is massive. Curiously, after the 2009 H1N1 debacle, an article was published on the NIH website titled "'Listen to the People': Public Deliberation about Social Distancing Measures in a Pandemic." The article notes the vital need for good and honest communication to the public about measures being taken the protect the citizenry. It states: "Public engagement in ethically laden pandemic planning decisions may be important for transparency, creating public trust, improving compliance with public health orders, and ultimately, contributing to just outcomes."[7]

Ya think? This is something at which Fauci and company dramatically failed. At one point, early in the pandemic, Fauci advised against face masks but later admitted he was telling this "noble lie" to slow the impact on material needs and hospital settings. Honesty was a not a key feature of this pandemic.

The report continues: "We conducted focus groups with members of the public to characterize public perceptions about social distancing measures likely to be implemented during a pandemic. Participants expressed concerns about job security and economic strain on families if businesses or school closures are prolonged. They shared opposition to closure of religious organizations, citing the need for shared support and worship during times of crises."[8]

It was all right there. It is on the website of the National Institutes of Health.

They ignored all of it.

The report concludes: "Social distancing measures may be challenging to implement and sustain due to strains on family resources and lack of trust in government."[9]

What a stark and terrible reminder that the institutions that prided themselves on public health damaged the public more than anything else. Your trust should be in the bedrock of our Constitution, not in some self-endowed title of "science."

CHAPTER 3

The Pandemic Response Is Run by Intrepid Specialists! WRONG.

Whose idea was it to lock us all inside, eating takeout, getting fat, and going crazy with our kids for months on end? If you guessed Dr. Anthony Fauci, you'd be right. Early on in the pandemic, Dr. Fauci, the head of the NIAID and the highest-paid federal employee in the history of the United States, seemingly wondered aloud: *Lockdowns worked for the CCP, why not for us?* But it wasn't always that way.

In an early 2020 interview with TRT World, Dr. Fauci lamented the use of lockdowns by the CCP to "limit the ability to travel freely of about 55 million people."[1] Within weeks however Dr. Fauci had done an about-face and recommended a two-week shutdown of the entire country in the month of March. That shutdown would be extended another forty days—and might be extended again.

I recall that fateful day in late March in a ceremony in the Rose Garden. Dr. Deborah Birx, another of the Team Apocalypse health overlords, declared that the lockdown was going to be extended. I tweeted that "Donald Trump just lost the election."

This shocked a lot of people. I was an early supporter of President Trump when he ran for office and a strong defender of him during his tenure as president, but I wasn't blind to demographics. If even 2 percent of the top age demographic stayed home in November 2020 because of Covid fears, Trump would lose.

The Holy Covid Trio Are Terrible at Their Jobs

I like to give people the benefit of the doubt. I frequently encourage my colleagues to find the kindest interpretation of what they see in the crazy world of Covid. One friend who was very close to the situation at the Trump White House conveyed to me his utter dismay at the ineptitude present in the Covid task force. I offered, "Perhaps they're just trying to find the best way to save face in a difficult situation." He replied: "No, Justin, these people are dumb. These people are very dumb."

Here are the main players involved with the early stages the pandemic:

- Dr. Anthony Fauci, director of the National Institute of Allergy and Infectious Diseases (NIAID) and the chief medical advisor to the president
- Dr. Deborah Birx, who served as White House Coronavirus Response Coordinator under the Trump administration
- Dr. Robert Redfield, director of the Centers for Disease Control and Prevention and the administrator of the Agency for Toxic Substances and Disease Registry from 2018–2021

These players had their hand in every aspect of the pandemic response, and their decisions impacted every industry on the planet.

There is not enough room in these pages to digest and dissect a play-by-play rehearsal of what these folks did, but the disastrous steps that they took can be seen in microcosm in how each one treated the mask debate.

Dr. Fauci Lied from the Start

From documents obtained through the Freedom of Information Act (FOIA), we can see the sly pattern of deception and lies with how Dr. Fauci treated the subject in the public emails versus the private emails.

First, we have correspondence between Dr. Fauci and Sylvia Burwell, former U.S. secretary of Health and Human Services under President Obama. She asks Fauci about a trip she is taking via plane and is wondering if wearing masks is a good idea, and this is Fauci's response:

> Masks are really for infected people to prevent them from spreading infection to people who are not infected rather than protecting uninfected people from acquiring infection. The typical mask you buy in the drug store is not really effective in keeping out virus, which is small enough to pass through the material. It might, however, provide some slight benefit in keep[ing] out gas droplets if someone coughs or sneezes on you. I do not recommend that you wear a mask, particularly since you are going to a ve[r]y low risk location. Your instincts are correct, money is best spent on medical countermeasures such as diagnostics and vaccines.[2]

As Fauci notes, masks are for people who are infected trying not to infect others. Also, masks really don't protect the wearer, and finally, the masks you get at the drug store don't do anything anyway.

Later policy and pronouncements by Dr. Fauci would flatly reject this line of thinking. Contrast that with the policies enacted *still*, and policies that might come back at any time as our government sees fit.

In an email exchange with Robert Geller, vice president of medical affairs at Family Health Center, we learn that Dr. Fauci was certain the virus spread via aerosols:

> Thanks for the note.... Use an N95 if you have them available. Transmission is similar to influenza: respiratory droplets and likely a bit more as aerosol than with influenza. People can transmit even when they are asymptomatic. No approved therapies; however, we are doing clinical trials on 're-purposed' drugs such as remdesivir.... Vaccine going into phase 1 trial in about 6 weeks, but will not be ready for at least 1.5 years.[3]

This would have a been a massive public admission. For the next two years the official story was that the virus spread primarily by larger droplets and not aerosolization. Droplets *might* be contained by masks. But that is not how the virus spreads, and Fauci knew it all along. Keeping that fact from the public was a big lie.

As late as April 2020, Dr. Fauci was downplaying the use of masks and recommended their use only in medical practice settings. As noted Dr. Fauci also called to keep the wearing of masks "voluntary."

Famously, in a March 8, 2020, interview on *60 Minutes*, Fauci laughed off the use of masks:

There's no reason to be walking around with a mask. When you're in the middle of an outbreak, wearing a mask might make people feel a little bit better, and it might even block a droplet, but it's not providing the perfect protection that people think that it is. And, often, there are unintended consequences—people keep fiddling with the mask and they keep touching their face.[4]

Later, Dr. Fauci would claim that he made such pronouncements as a "noble lie" to protect the supply of masks for medical personnel and first responders.[5] From the start, much of our pandemic response was led by a self-admitted liar.

In hindsight, none of the masking showed any significant difference in stopping the virus. It turns out that the virus is seasonal, and once it starts up it must run its course. You might as effectively put forth your puny arm to stop the Mississippi River as you would mask to stop an aerosolized viral respiratory pathogen during a pandemic.

Dr. Birx and Dr. Redfield Spew Nonsense on Masks

Those facts didn't stop our next harbinger of idiocy in the unfolding debacle: Dr. Deborah Birx. By the time the second wave during the summer of 2020 had subsided, Arizona had seen the same type of massive wave up and then down. Dr. Birx—in front of President Trump, no less—declared that the masks had done it!

Fortunately, Dr. Scott Atlas was there to correct her that time. He recounted to me how he contradicted Dr. Birx right then and there. "This had nothing to do with masks," he said to Trump and the gathered press.[6]

Nevertheless, Birx continued to push masks for the next two years.

Then there was Dr. Redfield, who famously testified in front of Congress that he thought the use of the mask was perhaps even a better solution than vaccines.[7] He would later recant that statement, but the temptation to use this physical object as a panacea was something that many of our leaders succumbed to.

CHAPTER 4

Fauci's Gain-of-Function Research Is a Conspiracy Theory! WRONG.

S hortly after the first cases of COVID-19 were identified in the United States, multiple revelations about the origin of the virus came out.[1] A working group was established to investigate potential origins of the virus from the Wuhan lab. Subsequent emails from FOIA requests revealed a panicked Dr. Fauci when articles asserted a man-made origin of COVID-19.

On the morning of February 1, after an article by Jon Cohen was published on Science.org titled "Mining Coronavirus Genomes for Clues to the Outbreak's Origins,"[2] Dr. Fauci shot off a quick email to Hugh Auchincloss—a big cheese at the NIAID.

> Hugh: It is essential that we speak this AM. Keep your cell phone on. I have a conference call at 7:45 AM with Azar. It likely will be over at 8:45 AM. Read this paper as well as the e-mail that I will forward to you now. You will have tasks today that must be done.
>
> Thanks,
> Tony

Auchincloss replied later that morning:

> The paper you sent me says the experiments were performed before the gain of function pause but have since been reviewed and approved by NIH. Not sure what that means since Emily is sure that no Coronavirus work has gone through the P3 framework. She will try to determine if we have any distant ties to this work abroad.[3]

The "P3 framework" refers to one of the beloved projects of Dr. Fauci: gain-of-function research. This model allows researchers to investigate and adapt viruses to make them more lethal and transmissible, thus anticipating potential threats to humanity should one of these viruses evolve on its own.

Senator Rand Paul of Kentucky has been instrumental in holding Dr. Fauci's feet to the fire on the implication of those FOIA-produced emails: COVID-19 may have been man-made and leaked from the lab in Wuhan—all of it supported by U.S. taxpayer dollars.

CHAPTER 5

Covid Spreads Only by Droplets in the Breath! WRONG.

From the early stages of the pandemic, fearmongering became a lucrative career. Exposure on daily news channels, especially CNN, became the bailiwick of numerous members of Team Apocalypse. Early on, research couched their recommendations in emotional terms rather than science. "I would be terrified of eating at a restaurant where there are people not wearing masks," admitted research scientist Jeremy Howard, who was very concerned about the spread of the disease by droplets. "We really have to hit them at the source."[1]

This notion that the virus was spreading because we were spitting on each other took hold of every epidemiologist. This was the primary evidence for almost every major non-pharmaceutical intervention (NPI). If you're not near each other, there's no reason why you should worry about getting infected. This assumption that respiratory "droplets" primarily spread Covid was questioned by very few. The CDC only recently admitted that the primary transmission of the virus is via aerosolization—fine invisible clouds of Covid that could remain in a room or area for minutes if not hours. Given the large transmission and case rates we have seen, this shouldn't come as a huge surprise.

And it didn't. Many knew this was the case from the beginning yet refused to confirm the fact to the general public. Was this one of Anthony Fauci's well-meaning noble lies? Toward what end? No; the admission would have meant a loss of societal control by these mandarins and hawkers of doom.

The implications of the truth are massive: you cannot really stop an aerosolized viral respiratory pathogen from spreading. Masks won't work. Plexiglass barriers at checkout stands won't work. Social distancing won't work. There are no "droplets" filled with the disease that can be blocked. The mechanism is breath itself.

The Myth of the Asymptomatic Viral Spreader

The "droplet" assumption was coupled with an even more drastic accusation that took on moral dimensions: anyone could be a viral spreader—whether they had symptoms or not. In the Jim Carrey movie *Dumb and Dumber*, Carrey's character wonders aloud about a new virus: "But I don't have any symptoms!" Jeff Daniels answers: "That's one of the symptoms!"

Which is the case with practically *every disease* you currently don't have or never will have, obviously.

It was this assertion that drove almost *everything* about this pandemic. Painting everyone as a potential spreader might be the single biggest mistake foisted on the world. Even Dr. Fauci admitted early on in the pandemic that asymptomatic spread had never been a primary driver of previous viral diseases, but that notion was quickly thrown into the memory hole.

If *anyone* can spread the disease without knowing it, then *everyone* must be feared. The top health officer of my own county in San Diego, Wilma Wooten, advised people in August 2020 to "assume that everyone has COVID-19."[2] She could be counted on again and again to instill fear in a population already confused as to who and what they should fear.

This was the perfect set of tools for our health overlords: Anyone can be a spreader. Better safe than sorry.

CHAPTER 6

Everyone Is at Serious Risk from Covid! WRONG.

Most people are lousy at estimating their risk for COVID-19 disease. One poll taken in 2021 noted that both Republicans and Democrats seriously overshot the chance of hospitalization and death from COVID-19. Nearly 30 percent of Democrats believed that one out of every ten people would die after contracting the virus. Half of Democrats (and a good portion of Republicans) believed that the hospitalization rate from getting sick with Covid was an order of magnitude larger than it is.[1]

As a general rule of thumb, you can simply check someone's birthdate for the most accurate means to assess his risk.

If the average age of death from the COVID-19 pandemic is eighty years old, then for every twenty years below that gauge your risk of dying of COVID-19 goes down ten times. So, if you are sixty years old, your risk is ten times lower than that of an eighty-year-old, and if you are forty years old, your risk is one hundred times lower than an eighty-year-old's. If you are twenty years old, your risk is one thousand times lower than your aged grandparents. If you are a child, your risk is literally *ten thousand times* lower.

Professor John Ioannidis, professor of medicine, epidemiology, and population health and expert in biostatics at Stanford, reckoned that if you are *under* the age of sixty-five your risks of dying of COVID-19 are about the same as your risks of dying from an annual commute to work on a weekly basis. If you are *over* the age of sixty-five, your risks are larger and akin to the risk of dying that a professional truck driver takes over the course of a year.[2]

Here in the United States about eight thousand people die every day. Forty thousand people die every month in nursing homes. Over the course of the pandemic, at the time of this writing, just over one million total deaths have been attributed to COVID-19 (we'll examine this claim later). Over that same two-year period from 2020 to 2022, about 6.5 million people have died of other causes.

The simple fact is that the rain falls on the just and the unjust. We all die. The average age of death for an American is between seventy-five and eighty years old. That also happens to be the average age of death of those dying from COVID-19. As you go down in age, the risk of dying from Covid doesn't just reduce dramatically, it falls as if you'd thrown the numbers off a cliff.[3]

Boomers Are Hundreds of Times More Likely to Die

Nearly 85 percent of all the deaths with Covid are people over the age of sixty. That age group makes up just 15 percent of the overall population. Now consider the 1918 Spanish flu. The average age of death for that pandemic was about twenty-eight years old. What if during the COVID-19 pandemic thousands of twenty-somethings, teens, and children were dropping dead every day? As it stands at the moment, the average number of children dead from Covid across all fifty states is forty-six. Forty-six *people*, not 46 percent.[4]

Any life at any age is worth saving, but the impact on society of someone dying at eighty years old is much different than the impact of a child who dies. One statistic that actuaries use to gauge the impact of a large mortality event is "Years of Life Lost" (YLL). Given that the average age of death in the United States is about eighty years old, if you die at the age of seventy-eight, that is two years of life lost. If a child dies of COVID-19, that is seventy-plus years of life lost. The loss of our loved ones at any age to a pandemic can be tragic, but the impact of losing a young child on a family and society at large is much different than the impact of losing an aged grandparent. This simple fact explains why the 1918 Spanish flu outbreak was massively more impactful when compared to the COVID-19 pandemic.

The Chance of Children Dying Is Almost Nonexistent

You can compare the risk of dying of COVID-19 compared to other causes of death to the overall population. How many people do you know who have *died* from choking on food or sunstroke? Yet those risks are similar to the risk of your dying from Covid in your twenties or thirties.[5] They are miniscule.

The initial claim given by the World Health Organization and China was that COVID-19 had a mortality rate of 3 percent or higher, that it was twice as deadly as the average seasonal flu.[6] Later, Dr. Fauci would claim in front of Congress that the mortality rate was 1 percent.[7] Both these figures are *vastly* overstated.

In 2020 we were a year away from the high impact 2017–18 flu season where there had been approximately 61,000 deaths and an estimated 44 million infections in the United States. That comes out to roughly *fourteen tenths of 1 percent* of the population. For every 10,000 people who got the flu in 2017–18, 14 would eventually die.[8] It turned out that the governmental interventions and mandates almost all stemmed from the unfounded fears brought about by core stats which were wholly misinterpreted.

Let's take up the grisly task of counting deaths over time. First, we need to bracket the onset of Covid in the United States, spring 2020, which was the most impactful stage of the pandemic and needs to be considered separately. So start in June 2020. Between June 2020 and February 2021, many parts of the nation were in lockdown mode. From June 2021 to February 2022, the vaccines were out and being given nationwide. Compare the two periods. The year 2021 saw a big rise in deaths in certain regions compared to the year before. Yet June 2021 to February 2022 show that the waves synced as we approached the winter. When you add it all up into a cumulative count of deaths you quickly realize there is little to *no difference*: about four hundred thousand deaths over each time period.[9]

It's an astounding realization. After all the non-pharmaceutical interventions, after the huge adoption of vaccines almost across the board—the masks, the social distancing, the mandate—after all the efforts to educate and change behavior, in the end none of it mattered. The virus was going to virus. There was no stopping it.

To sum up, your risk is probably relatively low. For the vast majority of people, COVID-19 is something you will survive just fine. The data that we do have is seriously lacking.[10] It will be years before we truly know the impact of COVID-19, but based on what we know, the data vastly overshot the actual deaths and societal burdens that have been touted by officials and the press.

CHAPTER 7

If You Die *with* Covid, Then You Die *from* Covid! WRONG.

Kary Mullis, the Nobel Prize–winning inventor of the PCR test, had some stark opinions on Tony Fauci. In an interview from the 1990s, Mullis said of Fauci: "Guys like Fauci get up there and start talking, you know, he doesn't know anything really about anything, and I'd say that to his face. Nothing."[1]

Mullis was particularly critical of Dr. Anthony Fauci's approach to the diagnosis of diseases. Much controversy surrounds Dr. Fauci and his efforts in the 1980s to deal with HIV/AIDS epidemic. Mullis continued: "The man thinks you can take a blood sample and stick it in an electron microscope and if it's got a virus in there you'll know it. He doesn't understand electron microscopy, and he doesn't understand medicine, and he should not be in a position like he's in."[2]

Certainly, the decision to use the extremely sensitive PCR-test array to find Covid viruses will go down as one of the worst decisions of the pandemic. By comparison, at the height of the pandemic, we were performing more tests to find Covid in an hour across the country than we perform to find influenza in an entire year. Testing regimes required a massive outlay of funding from the federal government. The initial amount allocated was $12 billion from the CARES Act passed by Congress but additional funding of $75 billion has been allocated for future testing. Based on these expenditures we will be testing Americans for Covid well into the next two decades.

PCR Tests Are Extremely Oversensitive

Every point of this industrial testing approach was approved under an emergency use authorization (EUA), which meant that certain steps, quality assurances, and standard operating procedures were streamlined or dropped altogether. Lab technician qualifications were shifted to address the volume of workers needed to deploy these systems. Huge financial windfalls were granted to companies willing to take a risk in this speedy environment. As we mentioned above, the cycle threshold settings were placed to capture the widest possible set of cases. Team Reality was lambasted for implying that a Covid case *wasn't necessarily* a Covid case, but by early 2022 even CDC director Rochelle Walensky had to admit that these tests were picking up cases with no live virus as late as twelve weeks after infection.[3]

The result was a massive quarantine of healthy people with few or any symptoms. This led to job losses and negative economic impact as mandates forbid on-site exposure until ten to fourteen days after the first positive test, and only a negative test would allow you back into the flow of life.

As a result there was huge overstatement of the number of people hospitalized for Covid. By one estimate 50 percent of all Covid patients were in the hospital for something else entirely.[4] Finally, there was a massive overcounting of Covid deaths based simply on a positive test result. In some states, deaths were counted as Covid deaths sixty days or even ninety days after recovery from Covid![5] If the person died within three months after a bout with Covid, well then, it was a fatality due to Covid.

This frightful wide net casting we discussed above hugely impacted morale across the country. As the pandemic waned in the spring of 2022, one report noted that 65 percent of all hospitalizations were *incidental* infections—people were in the hospital for something else, but because they tested positive for Covid, they were logged into the books as a Covid bed.[6]

Hospitals Cheat on Reporting

If the infrastructure of testing ensured a blurring of the notion "with Covid" versus "from Covid," then the financial incentive structure of hospitals put the Covid dashboards on tilt. The CARES Act passed Congress and was signed by President Trump in March 2020. This was the catch-all bill that eventually led to an outlay of $6 *trillion* to address the virus and the lockdowns. Part of that package was a generous reimbursement for hospitals. On average, a hospital would receive around $10,000 for a Covid patient and $39,000 for a Covid patient sent to the ICU. In rural areas, that reimbursement amount might be as high as *$90,000 per patient*.[7] With dollars behind each bed, there was no real incentive to be picky about "with" versus "from."

That's not to say that our hospitals in America are nefarious bilkers of taxpayer dollars (although, there is plenty of bilking), but put yourself in the shoes of a hospital administrator. One of the first mandates for hospitals in specific areas was to cancel "elective" surgeries. For many healthcare services, this is the most profitable part of their entire operation. What's more, the emergency rooms were not bursting at the seams as predicted. Ironically, ERs across the country would see the lowest level of visitors as people lived with injuries and sickness just to avoid Covid. Stopping and slowing down these operations led to many hospitals shuttering altogether. By the end of 2020, nearly 20 rural hospitals had closed for good across the United States, the highest yearly total in a downward trend that started in 2005.[8] Think on that: in an epidemic, hospitals were going out of business.

There Is Money to Be Made in Shoddy Covid Reporting

If you are a hospital administrator, it almost behooves you to maximize the reimbursement you receive from the government. As we see, it can mean the life or death of the institution. Indeed, in October 2020, government agencies overseeing reimbursement allowed hospitals to count observation beds with Covid patients as full inpatient Covid beds, leading to a seeming burst of admissions in late October right as fears grew for a rough Covid winter. Any administrator worth his salt might attempt to keep it ethical, but would also try to maximize these outlays to keep the hospital's doors open.

As Team Reality members sifted through Florida death certificates, they noted that at least 30 percent of these Covid deaths were suspicious. When an eighty-nine-year-old female dies from a broken femur after falling from a height, but she is classified as a Covid death, we have a problem—and it's not a glitch in the Matrix. Someone has lied.

Nosocomial is one of the new words we added to our vocabulary during the pandemic. It denotes an infection acquired in a healthcare setting. We don't know the numbers on this, but it's not altogether impossible that most hospitalized COVID-19 patients across the entire pandemic were *incidental* and transmitted in the hospital.

Ventilators Violate the Hypocritic Oath

Here's an outrage that quickly disappeared from the news. Early in the pandemic it was thought that hospital ventilators would be needed en masse to address growing respiratory conditions for ICU patients with Covid. Unfortunately, a very high percentage of those who are intubated die. The demand for these devices was so high that President Trump invoked the Defense Production Act to mandate the assembly of vents at a high pace output. Many doctors came to question the viability of doing so many intubations; then it was revealed through multiple interviews in the *New York Times* that those early intubations that were performed were done *not to help the patient breathe* but *to slow the spread of the disease to other staff and patients*. This is a deliberate violation of the Hippocratic oath.[9]

The top health overlords knew the data was bogus, but they let it go out regardless. There was no effort to qualify cases, hospitals, and deaths in any meaningful way. By the spring of 2022, numerous states were revising their death totals downward. From March 2022 to April of that same year, the CDC alone removed over 70,000 deaths from the case surveillance file.[10]

Mullis didn't mince words about these people:

> Most of those guys up there on the top are just total administrative people, and they don't know anything about what's going on in the body. You know, those guys have got an agenda, which is not what we would like them to have, being that we pay for them to take care of our health in some way. They've got a personal kind of agenda. They make up their own rules as they go. They change them when they want to. And they smugly—like Tony Fauci does not mind going on television in front of the people who pay his salary and lie directly into the camera.[11]

There Is a Massive Overcount

We have surpassed one million COVID-19 deaths according to the CDC.[12] By the summer of 2020, the team at Rational Ground was aghast at the wide-ranging and inaccurate data coming out of the official data feeds from the government. We knew that a cascade of awful errors was allowing Team Apocalypse to blow the stats out of proportion.[13] The PCR tests were so inaccurate that they could pick up a "positive" Covid case at five days after infection or even seventy-five days after infection. This fact alone was suppressed until late in 2021 when even Dr. Rochelle Walensky, the new head of the CDC, had to admit the sensitivity of the tests. This meant that many deaths being attributed to Covid had *no live virus* at the time of death, but because they tested positive, they were noted as Covid deaths regardless.

Furthermore, a large portion of the infections for Covid were infections that originated at a healthcare provider such as a hospital. With hospitals being the first point of care and a major hub of testing, the infections ran rampant among those who were patients at the hospital—even if they were there for something else altogether. Even Dr. Fauci had to admit that during the enormous wave of infections from the omicron variant many of these infections, especially among children, were incidental infections. They would never have occurred outside the healthcare setting.

Finally, hospitals and county coroners were instructed to use a wide latitude in tagging deaths for the Covid counts. This was something that happened across the country. In some instances a death could be counted as a Covid death even if the person was ninety days out from a positive Covid test.[14]

These factors along with many other complications ensured a likely massive overcount of Covid deaths across the world. One egregious example was that in March 2022 the CDC revised childhood

Covid deaths, reducing the totals by *one-fourth* of what had been previously reported because of a *clerical error*.[15]

Our health overlords are playing with a wide net when it comes to COVID-19 cases, hospitalizations, and deaths. Unfortunately for them they can't completely hide the rigging from the data-digging obsessives of Team Reality when the results come out the other end.[16]

Even on the sensitive subject of vaccine data, we know much is amiss. We noted that the CDC had been less than forthcoming in its export of valuable vaccine data. We know they have a lot more information than they currently reveal around vaccinations, hospitalizations, and mortality. They just don't want to share it.

Authorities and Institutions Are Lying on Purpose

In a February 2022 interview in the *New York Times*, "Kristen Nordlund, a spokeswoman for the CDC, said the agency has been slow to release the different streams of data 'because basically, at the end of the day, it's not yet ready for prime time.'"[17]

This was two years into the pandemic. There had been plenty of time to get the numbers right. "Not ready for prime time" was obviously code for "this data will make us look bad."

We saw the same political approach to health data obscurity being adopted in Scotland. Like most of the United Kingdom, Scotland has a single source of information with a nationalized healthcare system. During the first two months of 2022, data showed that vaccinated individuals were *more* at risk from omicron than unvaccinated individuals in many age demographics. To avoid the embarrassing data, Scotland just up and admitted they wouldn't put the data out there.

"Public Health Scotland will stop publishing data on covid deaths and hospitalisations by vaccination status—over concerns it is misrepresented by anti-vaxx campaigners," reported the *Glasgow Times*.[18]

In other words, they were suppressing the truth in order to serve a political purpose—and admitting that was exactly what they were doing, as if that condoned their censorship of data paid for by the very citizens they were maligning.

They Massage the Data

In the United States, multiple reports declare that the difference between vaccinated and unvaccinated individual's rates of getting the omicron variant is nearly 1000 percent. Upon closer investigation this rate is basically nonsense. The United States, the Centers for Disease Control (CDC), Health and Human Services (HHS), and the Food and Drug Administration (FDA) are using the wrong denominators, and in many instances vaccination records lag because they need to be matched to other systems.[19] To put it another way, when people come into hospitals for Covid treatment, unless their vaccination record is in that hospital's record system, that record would have to be manually matched by someone. In the meantime that person is given the status of unvaccinated, which then *widens* the gap of the final numbers when they publish.[20]

The government is bad at all of this. They hide the data and refuse to face the data they make public. They distract from this terrible record by lamenting the number still unvaccinated. Complaining about these problems won't bring back the certain dead from the un-jabbed masses, Team Apocalypse would say.

The truth is very different than the alarm bells they constantly ring. Over 80 percent of the at-risk population (those above sixty-five years old) are fully vaccinated. Close to 100 percent of the highest risk group (eighty years plus) are vaccinated.[21]

While Team Apocalypse is heavily invested in pushing the narrative of the anti-vax Trump voter, the easiest way to predict vaccine hesitancy is simple: age. If you're not at risk for the disease, then you probably aren't naturally motivated to go get the vaccine. The data shows that 99.995 percent of all COVID-19 deaths occurred in people over the age of fourteen. Similarly, 99.74 percent of deaths were among those older than twenty-five. And remember, nearly 80 percent of the Covid deaths occurred in people aged over sixty-five.[22] If you are young, even middle-aged, your chance of dying from Covid is exceedingly low, fading to almost nonexistent in the very young. No wonder many simply chose to skip the vaccine (which, of course, comes with its own risk).[23] It's an extraordinary feat of propaganda that the United States has gotten the overwhelming majority of adults to get vaccinated at all.

However, the pandemic plan hasn't panned out as Fauci and company thought it would, and the mixed messaging from previously trusted institutions—on issues, for example, like masking up the fully vaccinated—has caused irreparable harm.

CHAPTER 8

If You Don't Wear a Mask, You're Killing Grandma! WRONG.

One of my colleagues relates an incident he had on a local train ride into New York City. It was several months into the mask craziness in 2020. He had just grabbed his coffee and sat down across from another lady who grasped her own coffee tightly but was dutifully wearing her mask. As he approached his seat (his coffee cup not yet visible) the woman made a face of shock—or rather her eyes widened since he couldn't see the rest of her face—but he presumed correctly that it wasn't a smile. He was not (yet) wearing a mask. She grew pale until he brought his coffee cup into view and pressed it to his lips as he sat down across from her. At which point she too removed her mask to take a sip of her coffee. My friend thought, *I drink my coffee to protect you, you drink your coffee to protect me.* The perfect symbiosis of public psychosis and maddening health policy.

Frankly, as my wife notes, "Some people seem to really like it." And why wouldn't they? Our modern society rewards such virtue, and while the mask doesn't have the protective effect that some expect (even CNN contributors have deemed cloth masks "facial decorations"), it acts as a *talisman* of sorts.[1]

Masks Are Props in the Theater of the Absurd

Lest you think I exaggerate, one of the few mask studies published just before the pandemic admitted that the thin layer of sweaty, drool-soaked fabric probably isn't protecting anyone, but, the authors extoled, "It is also clear that the masks serve symbolic roles. Masks are not only tools they are also talismans that may help increase health care workers' perceived sense of safety, well-being and trust in their hospitals." They continue: "Although such reactions many not be strictly logical…"[2] Actually, let's stop there.

Not strictly logical?

A talisman?

I can handle a *lot* of nonsense from my elected officials, but I expect a little more from published, peer-reviewed, and accredited "experts" in the revered *New England Journal of Medicine*. I remember the Brady Bunch in Hawaii where the kids had a talisman. If I could wave a wand, I would keep that word enmeshed in the episode forever and probably ban it from any use in medical journals. Are we placating the gods of some volcano?

Do you remember the first time you saw a person wear a mask (that is, besides your mom's gynecologist as you made your way into this world)?

If you're over the age of twenty-five, you might have a recollection of the King of Pop doing so. Remember Michael Jackson with his entourage in tow, an umbrella handler, maybe a monkey (or was that Elvis with the monkey?), and MJ himself donning a black mask as he wandered past his fans and the paparazzi? Biographers say that he was a bit of a germaphobe and wore the mask to protect himself from getting sick.

Fast forward twenty years. Numerous entertainment rags during the pandemic wondered aloud "Did Michael Jackson Predict COVID-19?"[3]

Journalism has really taken a hit during the pandemic. Unfortunately, Covid hysteria came in at the very moment that online magazines hit a crossroads. Clickbait is the name of the game, and the virus spawned an entire industry of headlines, copycat articles, and social media sharing tactics that endure to this day. I count no fewer than twenty-four headlines declaring the clairvoyance of Michael Jackson. All of them seem composed from the same quote given by a former bodyguard: "He knew that a natural disaster was always there. He was very aware and would always predict that we could be wiped out at any time. That a germ that could spread."[4]

Now think again. When did you first learn that the flimsy piece of cloth you and your kids strapped on for two years was not to protect you the wearer but rather to protect those around you? Some of you might be learning this for the first time right now. The inconsistency of messaging is a massive failure of our health overlords.

Masks Are Mostly Virtue Signals

The evidence for masks in the healthcare industry has ebbed and flowed. There are numerous studies looking at the efficacy of masks in a medical ward, and almost all of them show little to no prevention of the transfer of respiratory illnesses. Rather, the masks are there for the close-up spittle of your dentist, doctor, hygienist, or (in the heightened atmosphere of 2022) even strippers.[5]

But let's ignore the stripper pole for the moment and return to dentistry. A dentist friend described to me his profession's OSHA-certification training process for masks. The personal protection equipment (PPE) specialist sits next to you, and you put on your surgical mask and go about your dental duties. One wrong move, one errant touch or adjustment of the mask with your fingers and—*slap*—they make you discard the mask and start over again. The folks at OSHA take their hygiene very seriously—until the CDC and the surgeon general came out with their recommendations on how to make your own mask at home from a T-shirt! OSHA embarrassingly stayed silent during most of the pandemic. Silent, that is, until it came time to force a needle into everyone's arms (more on that later).

How many times did you discard your mask during the pandemic? I'm guessing you did a lot of re-use. Ever have a spousal quarrel about using your wife's mask? How often did you misplace a piece of breathable cloth that was beloved because it was easier to gasp through?

Looking back we can all say in unison: Ew.

In short, Michael Jackson was wrong, and your dentist knows best. The regular surgical and cloth masks are not meant to protect the wearer—they're meant to protect the moaning person reclined in the chair waiting for the Novocain to kick in because a crown came loose.

This masking game has given an entire generation a moment to display their worthiness. We've never had the equivalent before: a visible, outward behavior that not only demonstrates one's virtue but whose absence denotes literal death—or rather intent to murder. Team Reality has received innumerable pronouncements during the pandemic on our potential to injure, maim, or kill grandma and children by refusing to mask up and encouraging others not to.

Welcome to the world of Covid where every virtue signal can be had for the price of a face diaper. You can wear it, use it to warn others, to berate others, or even to decorate your Christmas tree. Of course, when you apply a public policy across the board and create a new dynamic for every human interaction, the results are disastrous. Sometimes small—sometimes far reaching. Masks are a curse on society.

CHAPTER 9

Masks Are Imperfect but Keep Covid in Check! WRONG.

Working with Rational Ground writers, a group of parents in Gainesville, Florida, sent six face masks to a lab at the University of Florida, requesting an analysis of potential contaminants. The lab responded: "The resulting report found that five masks were contaminated with bacteria, parasites, and fungi, including three with dangerous pathogenic and pneumonia-causing bacteria." The analysis detected "dangerous pathogens on the masks." These included bacteria that cause:

- Pneumonia
- Tuberculosis
- Meningitis
- Amebic encephalitis
- Lyme disease
- Diphtheria
- Many, many others.[1]

"A parent who participated in the study, Ms. Amanda Donoho, commented: 'We need to know what we are putting on the faces of our children each day. Masks provide a warm, moist environment for bacteria to grow.'"[2]

There is likely cow herpes on your kid's mask as well.

By the end of 2021, the following points had all been confirmed in studies and the media. Even the vaunted lockdown proponents on CNN at one time or another conceded most of these points: Cloth masks don't work. Asymptomatic testing isn't effective. Closing schools doesn't prevent deaths. N95 masks aren't appropriate for kids. The vaccine doesn't stop the spread.

These findings are not new. We've known most of them throughout the pandemic.[3]

Masks Wearing Is a Cult

Every industry had its own unique fixture on the non-pharmaceutical interventions (NPIs). One correspondent relates:

> I work in the classical music industry and almost every moment is characterized by Covid madness and virtue signaling. Many theaters have vaccine mandates but all still require lateral flow tests then tests on site before entering the theater and then still have mask mandates for backstage. Some even require string and percussion players to remain masked throughout whilst wind and brass are playing away a few feet behind. Performing with an (unmasked) world famous violinist recently and another musician was required to put a mask on, during the performance, to move closer and turn pages. The lists of insanities are endless and endlessly wearing.

To review: By mid-2020 Americans were bound by a public policy endowing magical protections to a piece of cloth. The policy protected all wearers and gave permission for adherents to lambast and ostracize non-wearers all while the media cheered on and buoyed such tension for nearly two years.

This is a cult.

Masks Bring Out the Worst in People

Pew Research conducted a poll in early 2022 asking Americans what gave their lives meaning. Nearly half said family, 18 percent indicated that material well-being was a boon, but one in twenty people responded that Covid was the main factor that gave their life meaning. In fact, more people indicated that the pandemic was worth living for than those who valued their pets above all.[4]

Virtue signaling is the domain of those who have nothing else to live for. Really. Monuments were provided with masks and well-known sayings were given a Covidian makeover. Dan Rather, who never met a draconian measure he didn't love, tweeted "Mask not what your country can do for you. Mask is what you can do for your country."[5]

Holidays became a fond vehicle to demonstrate the fullness of Covid within you.[6] Other would denote their obeisance in selfies published to social media. "Going to keep wearing my mask on public transport," wrote one Brit, "even when it's just me on the tube." Her selfie confirmed that she was indeed alone on the Underground.[7]

Then we have all the virtue contained in the juicy goodness of a vaccine. Remember how the previous generation was a little bit shy about the scar left by the polio vaccine? Not this one. They want to remember it long after it fades. A myriad of Covid tattoos show arms clad in the ever-present spike-virus shape with the flavor and date of their vaccine shot. One read: "Pfizer, March 24, 2021."[8]

This obeisance to a corporate product in a *tattoo* is beyond ironic. It's just sad.

For many there was pressure to don the mask not just to demonstrate obeisance in real life but to apply it to all your social media avatars. This pressure to enjoin this iconography to your virtual self creates an instant grouping mechanism. When the mask fad started to fade, the virtue signaling searched for its next denotation—this time in the form of a vaccination. Syringes and official, blue-checked vaccinations adorned Facebook and Twitter icons. Even Tinder had the means to verify one's vaccination status!

Masks Are a Step toward Political Oppression

Masks, lockdowns, and vaccine mandates manifested a trio of seemingly unassailable virtues during the height of the pandemic. They still do. Demonstrating good character isn't just a self-satisfying gesture—in many social circles it was a requirement for entry, sometimes literally for freedom itself. In some countries your outward gestures to the cult of Covid were considered sacrosanct, even obligatory—the punishment was internment. *You must demonstrate this virtue; otherwise we will cut you off and send you to jail.*

In New Zealand and Australia, internment camps were built to house those infected—most of whom were no doubt a passel of Covid lepers who refused masking. This all seemed to be going hunky-dory until Covid caught up with the rest of the populace. As our colleague Ian Miller has documented, since the awe-inspiring lockdowns of the great Down Under, cases have grown several thousandfold.[9]

CHAPTER 10

Plexiglass Barriers in Stores and Businesses Save Lives! WRONG.

Back in 2020 it was presumed that the massive wave of cases blasting across the country were caused primarily by droplets spewing out of people's orifices and landing on other people. It would take another twenty months before it was generally conceded that SARS-CoV-2 was an aerosolized viral respiratory pathogen—in which case the microscopic particles could simple waft above or through any new apparatus and dance about in the air as if there were no barrier at all. Because there wasn't one for them.

Take plexiglass, for example. Someone at the CDC decided that what we needed more than anything else to stop the spread of Covid in retail stores and schools was a ubiquitous deployment of plastic barriers. The National Grocers Association polled its members in the summer of 2020 and found that 84 percent of respondents had put up plastic shields in their stores.[1] The International Association of Plastics Distribution recorded revenues that were up significantly compared to 2019. For most of America however, every grocery store, gas station, DMV, and school now resembled a check-cashing joint from the inner city.

Home Depot took it a step further. Massive metal mounts with plexiglass separated cashiers from the customers. I guess if you're Home Depot that's the way to do it. Why not? You have everything right there.

What has gone undiscussed is that the CDC very quietly and without any particular notice *dropped* their recommendation of plexiglass from their retail recommendations. Several studies materialized demonstrating that creating more surfaces to clean and maintain probably isn't helping. Another study noted that plastic barriers impede the flow of ventilation—stagnant air being one of the few proven methods to keep the plumes of Covid hanging around in a room.[2]

But consider those tens of millions of dollars spent to erect these plastic barriers, not to mention the strained vocal cords of millions of Americans trying to speak through a mask and then through a plastic barrier. Customer: "I'd like to buy some stamps." Cashier: "I'm sorry. I'm married. I won't dance with you."

Lastly, very few discussions are being had about the waste by-products we are producing during the pandemic. Recall that some grade schooler back in 2011 came up with the science campaign declaring the dangers of plastic beverage straws. Since that time the world must bear up with the completely unnecessary replacement of plastic straws with paper straws. Paper straws react to the liquids just as you would expect. Metal straws had been a popular compromise until some unsuspecting woman in England died after impaling her eye on a metal straw while tripping.[3]

A report from the WHO in February 2022 noted that approximately 87,000 tonnes of personal protective equipment were produced and procured over the course of the pandemic until that time (a tonne equals about 1.1 tons). Most of it will end up as waste. It doesn't stop there. They also found:

- 140 million test kits generating 2,600 tonnes of waste
- 731,000 liters of chemical waste
- 144,000 tonnes of waste from syringes, needles, and safety boxes[4]

I would pay good money to witness Greta Thunberg dress down Dr. Fauci over this atrocious crime perpetrated on the environment. But I won't hold my breath. Of course, if I were to hold my breath, both Greta and Tony would be greatly pleased considering that, according to them, what I exhale will kill the planet and every grandma I encounter.

CHAPTER 11

Keeping People Inside and Locked Down Saves Lives! WRONG.

Early on the Science and Technology Directorate at the Department of Homeland Security was given rare access to captured particles of the SARS-CoV-2 virus itself. Upon experimentation the S&T noted that the virus is almost completely destroyed at the slightest exposure to direct sunlight.[1] When they gave their briefing alongside Dr. Birx and Dr. Fauci, I sensed that both of these top health leaders seemed disappointed. After all, if sunlight kills the virus, then the safest place for people to take refuge from the virus is outside. This notion was echoed a few weeks later during one of the morning briefings by then governor Andrew Cuomo of New York, who noted that 66 percent of new infections were occurring in home. He looks back at his screen to make sure he read that right. "This is surprising."[2]

One stark photo from the stay-at-home months shows a man on a beach in Southern California meditating. He is surrounded by eight police officers.

"Why are you here?" they ask. "Don't you know there's a stay-at-home order?"

The man chooses silence as they continue to rouse an answer from him. Outside. Sitting peacefully in sunlight.[3]

As numerous studies have shown, lack of vitamin D and obesity are two of the stark risk profiles for a potentially serious illness if you contract COVID-19.[4] Looking at the fully masked police officers around the man who sits cross-legged in a familiar meditation pose, one cannot help but comment that he is the only person in the picture not struggling with obesity. Of all the individuals on the beach that day, his risk was probably the lowest.

To date there is not a single confirmed case of outdoor transmission of COVID-19. Our health overlords could not bring themselves to allow the population a bit of freedom. Instead, they locked people into homes where the infection was already present, ensuring that everyone in the household would get the disease.

CHAPTER 12

Vax Mandates Save Lives! WRONG.

Many Americans do indeed know their risks and no longer trust the government or government-beholden institutions to guide them. Vaccine mandates became a sore and important subject as 2021 ended. In typical fashion, the government flipflopped. Dr. Fauci declared in August 2020 that he didn't think mandates would come around.[1] We at Rational Ground predicted that he couldn't resist the authoritarian urge for long.[2]

We were right.

But why should Americans mind vaccination mandates? After all, we have vax mandates for children in schools already! This is another tactic thrown at us by Team Apocalypse. They declare: Polio, measles, and MMR vaccines are already required! Our response is simple: The mandates for these vaccines came years (six to sixteen years) after the vaccines had been fully approved. We have *never* mandated a vaccine that's less than a year old.

Covid Vaccines Are Unknown Territory for Kids

The coming wave of new data around vaccinations may not be very pretty. Some serious concerns are currently being raised about the impact on young children. If you've been infected with COVID-19 previously and recovered, your antibody titers are pretty robust (titers are a measure of your immune system's antibodies to ward off Covid). The younger you are, the more robustly those titers are sustained. Recent data uncovered from Pfizer suggests that if person is vaccinated after having recovered from COVID-19, those titers can go tilt like a pinball machine and form immune complexes within the body that could cause problems. For instance, our Rational Ground colleague, analyst Jean Rees, found younger people had moderate to severe joint pains after vaccinations.[3]

In March 2022, based on this and other information, the Florida Department of Health, under the direction of state surgeon general Joseph Ladapo, officially recommended against giving coronavirus vaccines to healthy children. This was a controversial move to be sure, but the evidence of serious risks has been growing since the end of 2021. These types of adverse reactions are a point of much contention.

The federal government has played a duplicitous role in limiting further information on this topic. A database called the Vaccine Adverse Event Reporting System (VAERS), maintained by the CDC, allows for self-entry of adverse reactions from vaccines. This has been a deep controversy as adverse events are self-reported but typically submitted by a healthcare professional. The CDC has been a very hypocritical in addressing the use of VAERS. In one article they downplay the accuracy of the data of VAERS (which currently show tens of thousands of deaths attributed to COVID-19 vaccines) and then turn around the next week and use the very same data to bolster their policies on mask usage or such.[4]

Unlike the government, we on Team Reality recommend that you should, as always, make your own decisions about the vaccines. But the evidence against giving the current CDC-recommended doses to children is mounting.[5]

Millennial Deaths May Be Related to Vaccines

It's very possible that when all is said and done millennials will take a *big* grunt of the unexpected early deaths due to vaccines. It is still unclear why, but drug overdoses, depression, and unknown impact of vaccinations might be to blame. Specifically, for Americans between the ages of twenty-five and forty-four, there were 103,000 excess deaths for two years starting March 2020. As our colleague Ed Dowd notes, this is the equivalent of two Vietnams for this age group. Devastating.[6]

"Long Covid" Is Not Exclusive to Covid

One point of concerted pushback against vaccine mandates has been around the notion of so-called "long Covid." We on Team Reality take this with a grain of data-centered salt. The denotation covers a host of maladies affecting those who have seemingly recovered from Covid but still experience the ailments of having suffered the disease. From loss of smell to Covid toe, a host of challenges surround those who have survived.

Here is a litany of some of the consequences post-Covid:

- Acute ground glass opacity (NIH)
- Lung tissue damage (Science Daily)
- Chronic fatigue (Medical News Today)
- Neurological issues (*Journal of Neuroscience*)

- Cardiomyopathy (NIH)
- Ongoing symptoms and complications (CDC)
- Other long-term sequelae (CDC)

I fibbed a bit here. These are actually the documented post-recovery ailments associated with *regular influenza*.[7] As Akiko Iwasaki (an immunologist at the Yale School of Medicine) says, "While there's no doubt long Covid is a real condition worthy of diagnosis and treatment, this isn't unique to Covid."[8]

Does this mean there is no such thing as "long Covid"? Of course not. But aside from the loss of smell and taste there are no symptoms *exclusive* to Covid. It is a respiratory virus, and the impact is the same as almost every other pathogen. The relative newness of the virus is what sets it apart.

COVID-19 was overblown from early in the pandemic. The tests were overly sensitive, the fearmongering was massive, the infections at the hospital were not insignificant. The counting of Covid deaths was abhorrently done, and the vaccination numbers are deeply untrustworthy.

CHAPTER 13

Natural Immunity Is Not an Alternative to Vaccination! WRONG.

Health professionals began to speak up at the end of 2020 about "natural immunity," something that had been the mainstay of epidemiology for a century. To wit, if you get sick with the disease and recover, you likely have some form of strong immunity from getting it again. In 2004 Dr. Fauci was interviewed live on C-SPAN and was asked about someone who had already been diagnosed with influenza. The host of the program queried, "Should this person get the flu shot?" Dr. Fauci replied: "No, if she got the flu for fourteen days she's as protected as anybody can be...the best vaccination is to get infected yourself."[1]

Seemingly ignoring or even denying this probability, officials lambasted anyone who dared mentioned "natural immunity" as possessing a "let her rip" attitude—someone who wants to let the infection spread "willy-nilly," as one commentator put it.[2]

More insidiously, behind the scenes Dr. Fauci, Francis Collins (director of the NIH), and other officials were working to quell a group of academics who had produced a strong rebuttal to the prevailing Fauci regime called the Great Barrington Declaration. The

GBD, as it became known, was a consensus asserting that focused protection was a better approach than one-size-fits-all full lockdowns. The founders, Dr. Jay Bhattacharya, Dr. Sunetra Gupta, and Dr. Martin Kulldorff, were derided in these emails as "fringe epidemiologists," and plans were put in motion to eliminate their influence. Natural immunity was the primary target.

Of Course Natural Immunity Can Be Acquired for Covid

What we can say almost for certain now is that if you had Covid and recovered, your immune system has all the tools it needs to combat the disease going forward. Marty Makary from Johns Hopkins University put it this way: "During every month of this pandemic, I've had debates with other public researchers about the effectiveness and durability of natural immunity," he wrote in an op-ed for *U.S. News & World Report* in August 2021. "I've been told that natural immunity could fall off a cliff, rendering people susceptible to infection. But here we are now, over a year and a half into the clinical experience of observing patients who were infected, and natural immunity is effective and going strong. And that's because with natural immunity, the body develops antibodies to the entire surface of the virus, not just a spike protein constructed from a vaccine."[3]

Natural Immunity Is Clearly an Alternative to Vaccination

One of the goals Rational Ground is *still* aiming to achieve is to get the government and other entities to recognize prior immunity as an alternative to vaccination or useless testing credentials.[4] The fact is that our national and state leaders in this time of crisis failed miserably and continue to deny even the most basic tenets of basic epidemiology.

You might say they lost their ever-loving minds, but that would be putting too nice a face on it. Their response has been one of deliberate deception, and it followed what became a worn path of repetitive actions:

They made up the Covid rules.
They ignored the negative impacts.
They overlooked conflicting data.
They demonized heterodox experts.
They censored research.
They disregarded control groups.
They acted surprised when the rules failed.
They claimed they had no idea.

PART 3

THE DAMAGE
TO CHILDREN

CHAPTER 14

Children Are Resilient and Will Bounce Back! WRONG.

Scientists have long studied the phenomenon that we all experience in which time seems to move slower when we are young and speed up as we age. We tend to remember specific days from our teenage years that lasted forever—either from pleasure or pain. Experts on neurology surmise that the brain is making new paths of memories as we experience things for the first time and thus the impression on the brain is seared into your mind quite literally.

What happens when you interrupt that natural flow of life and innocent acquisition of new experience? What if a massive portion of your youth is massively disrupted? The patterns of learning, experiences, milestones, achievements, opportunities are suddenly shut down. Think about the timing of this pandemic. While the two-year time frame roughly covers this crazy historic moment for adults, for our children it was three or more years. If your child started their high school freshman year in 2019, consider this:

- Schools closed across the country for the rest of the school year.

- A majority of schools did not reopen for his sophomore year until late into the spring in many states.
- His junior year was seriously disrupted with late starts and rolling quarantines that persisted into 2022.
- His senior year will start depleted of any major high school experiences. Few proms, few sporting events, no trips across the country, no trips abroad, few work opportunities, and lots of time with the family, at home.

The CDC reports that 55 percent of high school students reported emotional abuse by parents. The number of emergency room visits for suspected suicide attempts rose by 51 percent among teenage girls. Forty-four percent of children over the age of thirteen reported persistent sadness in their lives.[1]

Families Are Separated and Torn Apart by Government and Institutions

From my own experience with a mixed family, things were challenging. Stay-at-home orders limited our time together with one son, as he lives with his mother an hour north of me. Months went by before I could see him, his sister, and others outside my immediate circle. A year would go by before I would see my parents, before they could see their grandkids.

My stepdaughter was in her sophomore year of high school. I remember at the time feeling badly for the juniors and seniors of her small private school who would never get those choice upperclassman experiences. The grade schoolers and high schoolers were physically kept apart, depriving these young kids of mentorship and role models.

My stepdaughter garnered a very high score on the SATs and had some great prospects for schools in our state. Alas, a judge in

California ruled that the SAT scores could not be used for admissions because of the pandemic and the *unfairness* of the situation. Why did we spend all that time and effort on testing again? The admissions game for the years of the pandemic did not bode well for anyone. Massive waves of students took a "gap year" if they graduated in 2020, which meant that the 2021 college enrollment scene was pure chaos.

Again, had the sacrifices and loss of opportunities been balanced with a supported set of data showing that the measures taken reduced illness and deaths, children and parents might concede that it was worth it. If the ages of impact for COVID-19 had mirrored that of the 1918 Spanish flu, and tens of thousands of children had been felled by the disease, we might be having a very different conversation.

Instead, for our health overlords during Covid, it seems that children came last.

The impact on teens is palpable. They can articulate it to us. They can work through it in therapy. They can show regret and show courage to bear with these burdens. They are nearly adults, after all.

The impact on our small children is inexcusable.

Kids Cannot Defend Themselves and Have Been Deeply Harmed

As of this writing, the only people still in masks in a public school setting are preschoolers. The theory behind this abuse is awful. These children have not received authorization for the Covid vaccine and thus, in the minds of misinformed leaders, are vectors of disease and vulnerable. Initially, the CDC had reported over one thousand children dead from COVID-19. After much pushback, that figure was revised significantly and the number of deaths for preschoolers was very, very low. When you examine the CDC data on the underlying causes of death you realize quickly that these are incidental deaths and not attributable to Covid at all.[2]

Yet the damage is done. The developmental losses are massive, reports of a 300 percent increase in speech-therapy enrollments in one state, massive developmental losses in another.[3] These formative years cannot be replaced.

When the California state licensing board sat down with school leadership, they admitted that masks and distancing would definitely impact kids negatively. *But we have to do it. Those are our orders.*

We *have* to do it. We're just following orders.

The systems we trusted to protect our children have failed us.

Another preschool director told me that they would take turns calling in sick with Covid so that when the licensing folks called for a visit they would be scared off and reschedule the visit. Parents learned very quickly that fibbing to the school was the only way to keep their kids in school at all. It used to be that if you extended a vacation for your kids or wanted to take them out for the day you'd simply call in and say they were sick. Now, the fibs are reversed. If your child came down with a cold or was out because he wasn't feeling well (because, shocker, kids get sick with all sorts of things), you'd call it a personal day for the child. Otherwise, multi-day testing was required, and if the test came up positive for Covid, the entire class would be sent home. When society makes liars of parents to ensure their kids are treated well, society is broken.

CHAPTER 15

Children Are Walking Vectors of Disease! WRONG.

I try to reserve my ultimate wrath and judgement for those individuals and institutions that do real harm—especially to vulnerable children. Unfortunately, they are too many to enumerate individually, so I'm just going let loose and dish it out to everyone and anyone who made life unbearable for me or my kids—or tried to. In some cases below, I also dish it out to those entrepreneurial-minded inventors who were just trying to make the best of an awful situation. You made it worse instead.

Companies Treated Children as Lepers

Look, it's a young girl prancing into the front doors of her school. She waves, and I can only assume she is happy because she skips into the room.

This is a promo for a wonderful new product.

Even though this product is designed to replace a mask, our young protagonist is actually *still* wearing one underneath the thing. What thing?

Imagine a large plastic shield that encompasses a child's entire head. Imagine it's *your* child, going to school wearing a large plastic licorice jar on her head. The apparatus allows her to see (even though she is still wearing a mask underneath). The entire device is mounted to her chest with a Velcro strap around her back to ensure it remains fixed.

Imagine you're the insane engineer who looked at masks and plexiglass and decided, "Hey, let's put those two amazing things together!" The intention of the product is obviously to remove any chance of the spittle leaving her mask-clad mouth and landing on the person in front of her.

The teacher is wearing one too.

The advertisement declares that the product weighs less than one pound! This is meant to amaze us.

Next a teacher is seen inside the trapezoid terrarium. No doubt she could spend every waking moment in there, and it certainly seems like she could grow something below her chin where the fitted plastic meets her chest and shoulders. She smiles. Per usual, there is no mask on the adults.

"No Headaches, No Fogging, No Waste," the ad proclaims.[1]

This hellscape promotion comes from the good folks at Preferred Protective Equipment. In August 2020, given that masks were going to be part of our everyday lives, they decided to design an apparatus that still haunts me to this day.

One product allowed you to upload a picture of your child's smiling face. The company would then print the smile onto a mask adjusted directly to your child's chin. "Let them see you smile!" declared the banner ad. "Are you heading back into the classroom? Don't let your mask hide the joy of learning!"[2] The creepy, constantly smiling face was eerily reminiscent of some Batman villain. I'm certain any teacher would derive nightmares if a kid donned one in their classroom.

Infected Kids Are Stigmatized and
Categorized as Outcasts

One college put a prioritization around the dangers to students. It instructed its students in a pecking order of evacuations should a fire prompt an emergency. Students who were self-isolating after a positive Covid test were asked to let others evacuate first. After all, they might pass along Covid while perishing in the flames.[3]

A benign but equally upsetting incident occurred at a formal prom for a school dance. Masks were worn the entire time, but to ensure that no fluids were accidently passed teen to teen, the couples were asked to slow dance back-to-back.

The Kingston Trio could rightly sue for copyright infringement— this was indeed the zombie jamboree, "back-to-back, belly-to-belly." Couples linked arms with their backs to each other and awkwardly tried to sway back and forth. Dancers bumped into each other. Some tried a sly three-step. Everyone laughed. They laughed, but inwardly cringed.[4]

In Chicago schools the suspicion of disease vectoring burst to new levels. A *Washington Post* article described a "care pod being installed in Bell Elementary on Chicago's North side. Chicago Public Schools said that as a supplement to care rooms, a small fraction of our schools have been provided with care pods as a contingency safety measure."

The photo shows four upright, vertical chambers stretch across the stage, each one roughly the size of large telephone booth. Transparent plastic walls and ceiling make each pod an encased tomb, but thankfully an air filtration system blows fresh air into each via a set of air-conditioning tubes. All of this would serve just four students.[5] Bubble boy has been a running joke since the 1960s, but this misbegotten tech monstrosity takes it to new levels.

Kids Are Reduced to Mere Infection Risks

Several families took it upon themselves to film and upload videos of the most depressing and unnecessary scenes. Typically, this would involve young grandchildren aching to see their grandparents. A ghost-like aged figure would appear from a house draped in a plastic curtain or some other ridiculous barrier. The figure of the grandparent would then reach out to their kin in an awkward hug. So close, but never touching. The lessons taught to our children, that they are unredeemable points of infection, will not be lost on this generation as they come of age. It's an unnecessary travesty.[6]

CHAPTER 16

School Closures Are a Necessary Step to Save Lives! WRONG.

The fragility of our schools and education system has been exposed. Our Rational Ground colleague AJ Kay lamented the knee-jerk reaction of her special needs child's private school in November 2020: "My autistic daughter's private school—the one I transferred her to so she could resume the in-person instruction she so desperately needs—just closed for two weeks due to one reported case of #COVID-19."[1]

The whole school. One case.

Teachers Became Fearmongers and Terrible Examples

The fear of disease became contagious itself. Many teachers got caught up in the fearmongering. Some groups didn't feel that the schools were doing enough to clean and prepare. One teacher lamented on Twitter: "Our PreK team was told to report to school today. They will be cleaning their rooms while teaching remotely today. We provided our own PPE & cleaning supplies as our district…did not."[2]

The teacher provided photos to go with the tweet of the teachers in near hazmat-like suits with arms full of disinfectant wipes and cleaning supplies. Desks were spaced six feet apart with fixed, permanent plexiglass to boot. Some classroom rearrangers feared desks altogether and got rid of them. Teachers would presumably ply their trade in creative stations on the ground or carpet. One independent Alaska website stated, "Some of the youngest students returning to classes today in Anchorage will enter a dystopian classroom world, where they must kneel for hours on end on the floor while masked, and have no recess or art or physical expression."[3]

In Minneapolis the teachers' unions were so fearful they refused to go back to in-person learning until well into 2021. They set up "virtual learning centers" "where students are assisted by in-person staff in a room of similar size, ventilation, and ability to physically distance as a classroom." Teachers are in another room or at home altogether—teaching the kids *who are physically in the classroom* with laptops assisted by non-teaching staff. As our friend Matt Malkus noted on Twitter: "It only makes sense if you don't think about it."[4]

Children at one elementary school in Minnesota practiced the "zombie walk" with hands outstretched to keep a safe distance from other students and avoid touching anything on their way to lunch.

In other school districts, accommodations were made with a rotating schedule. Fearful concern was foisted on choir and band classes. One high school chose to have only three band students at a time come in on a three-week schedule. One mom posted a picture with only two students showing up and lamented: "How can you have a band with only 2 students? I'm afraid for the future of performing arts in public schools."[5]

One band teacher was taken aback by new school policies allowing kids back in the classroom. He wrote to parents that he was not yet ready for the students. "As a result of not expecting this situation," he wrote to parents, "I do not have preparations for masked band tomorrow and as a result we will need to cancel. It very much pains me to make this decision but I will be asking the school to provide me a couple boxes of surgical masks so I can cut slits and we can try it out next week."[6]

Pictures of band members playing with sliced masks for their wind and brass instruments filled the Internet. Other band practices continued with makeshift personal plastic tents for each band member. It was absurd and everyone knew it, but no one, it seemed, was empowered to change anything.

School Districts Destroyed the Very Possibility of Education

Many states doubled down on masking—literally. One school district in spring 2021 wrote parents: "We will require students to double mask after Spring Break.... This will ensure the safest environment possible as more students are in the classrooms."[7]

Some school districts would incentivize children to help on other programs with the reward...of breathing. In Florida, one school was conducting a shoe-and-sock donation drive. They wrote home to parents: "5th period won our class competition and will receive a 30 minute mask break tomorrow to celebrate, 5th period took 2nd place and will have a 25 minute mask break, and 2nd period took 3rd place and will have a 20 minute mask break."[8]

Other districts tried the reverse effect, punishing students if they misbehaved and taking away their mask breaks. The first point of misconduct would be to put the child in time-out. A second infraction would be a call home. The third infraction was the removal of the child's mask break.

The fear of Covid rose to drastic levels, and mask compliance became a means to let loose one's ire against the panic. In May 2021 a video of a bus driver in Colorado went viral after he slapped a student's face for refusing to wear a mask.[9] Lest we think this man crazy, consider that a large swath of the world truly believed that if you didn't wear a mask it was tantamount to murder.

Museums and Cultural Repositories Went Out of Their Way to Punish Kids

As the vaccines rolled out, pandemic fear found another excuse to fixate on children as a vector of disease. Museums, theaters, and other public venues made vaccines a mandated requirement for entry. Of course, for children the approval of vaccines wouldn't be had until well into the fall of 2021. One mom wrote in distress on Twitter: "My son, Leo, now age 10, at the Metropolitan Opera, which now forbids entry to those under 12 until they're vaccinated. Thank you...for denying a cultural pleasure to children. Thank you for doing your part running NYC into the ground and for declaring your fear of kids."[10]

A concerned mother and daughter wrote to Rational Ground about her situation: "My in-laws will now have not seen their grandchildren for two years because they are afraid. They are afraid to see us because our family is not vaccinated and the children, 12 & 15, will not be at any point. My in-laws are both fully vaccinated themselves. They are addicted to media fear porn and clearly do not trust the product they took yet will never admit that. I am at the point where they will be told they risk losing their grandchildren. I won't withhold them, but the kids will be busier as they mature and will move on with their lives."

As of this writing, kids are the last bastion of society still fully masked in many instances. Vaccine mandates are lifted, retail mandates for masking are lifted, but we still mask three- and four-year-olds with vigor. These same preschoolers take naps during the day. Do they mask when lying next to each other, lying still for two hours and sleeping? No—that would be dangerous.

CHAPTER 17

Lockdowns Keep Kids Alive! WRONG.

HealthDay reporter Robert Preidt noted a horrible trend in the summer of 2021: "Child Drownings in U.S. Pools, Spas on the Rise." Can you guess the cause? Here's a quick walk through:

Lockdowns -> Parents lose jobs -> Lack of income -> Schools closed -> Pools closed -> No swim lessons = More child drowning deaths than Covid deaths.[1]

A massive study out of Europe in April 2022 noted that the stringency of lockdowns and NPIs across various countries showed no measurable impact against the backdrop of serious Covid illnesses and deaths.[2] Studies in the United States also came to the same conclusion: there is precious little evidence that lockdowns, quarantines, stay-at-home orders, mask mandates, and public gathering strictures provided any beneficial relief on a state or county level. Careers were ended, schooling fractured, families upended, health destroyed, and reputations sullied all for naught.

Lockdowns Harm and Often Kill Children

A study in early 2022 from the World Bank, UNESCO, and UNICEF demonstrated how incredibly harmful the lockdowns had become. The school shutdowns were intended to "slow the spread" of the disease, but their result was instead to slow the minds of the children they impacted. The study estimated that about one and a half *billion* children had been forced to stay home due to school closures and education interruptions.

Young children with disabilities, poorer communities, and under-privileged backgrounds suffered the most. In Brazil, the report notes, "students learned only 28 percent of what they would have in face-to-face classes, and the risk of dropout increased more than threefold." In more rural areas like Karnataka, India, "the share of grade three students in government schools able to perform simple subtraction fell from 24 percent in 2018 to only 16 in 2020."[3]

Other studies noted the impact on students here in the United States. One research firm called Amplify noted: "In kindergarten, the percentage of students at greatest risk for not learning to read rose from 29 percent in the middle of 2019–20 to 37 percent in the middle of 2021–22." They go on to note that "48 percent of Black grade 1 students are far behind, and 43 percent of Hispanic grade 1 students, compared to 27 percent of white grade 1 students."[4]

This isn't just about short-term education loss; the evidence is pretty clear. Models can predict with some accuracy how degraded learning can impact a child's life well into the future. NWEA, a non-profit testing company, discussed these implications in a recent study showing "a 9 to 11 percentile point decline in math achievement (if allowed to become permanent) would represent a $43,800 loss in expected lifetime earnings. Spread across the 50 million public school students currently enrolled in grades K to 12, that would be over $2 trillion."[5]

The impact that this pandemic, the lockdowns, and the school closures will have on this generation will be massive.

CHAPTER 18

Teachers and Schools Were Hardest Hit by the Lockdowns! WRONG.

In 2021 the federal government authorized $122 billion in stimulus funds under the title "ESSER III," also known as "Elementary and Secondary School Emergency Relief," allocated under Title 1 monies. Ninety percent of the funding is intended for local districts. These school districts have three years to spend the money.[1] Disclosures of these funds are made public by the states, but there are lots of places to hide in the nooks and crannies—especially if no one cares to challenge education funding—which they don't.[2]

Covid Money Funding Years of CRT and Social Engineering in Schools

Schools are using some of the Covid government funds to re-engage with students. Numerous districts have big plans for getting students caught up.[3] Now there's a new source of perpetual Covid government largesse to look out for: the Build Back Better bills. And there is no better place to trace that movement than the school districts looking to amp up their infrastructure budgets.[4]

Reading over these detailed budget allocations, it's clear that Covid will reshape our entire education system, providing a massive opportunity and funds for forces intent on inserting themselves into our kids' education. Critical race theory proponents, school equity officers...you name it. The Great Reset has received an almost unimaginably large cash infusion.

Recall that the teachers' unions fought tooth and nail to keep our schools closed. Is it possible that they eked out this massive treasure for their own purposes in exchange for dropping their demands of "safety" at the school?

Remote Learning Here to Stay

Lastly, you can see from the massive monies assigned to "remote learning" (see this chapter's endnotes for details) that schools truly do anticipate more shutdowns to come. Perhaps some are even angling for them.

In his extensive study of learning loss across the decades, Eric Hanushek, a senior fellow at the Hoover Institution at Stanford University, has indicated that the earnings of kids who grew up in these pandemic years could be 6 percent to 9 percent lower than previous generations.[5] Loss of learning isn't something you can just catch up on. Masks, social distancing, quarantines, distance learning...we owe this generation a great deal for the harm inflicted them.

CHAPTER 19

School Reopenings Have Been Gradual but Effective! WRONG.

Many families feared schools would not reopen at all. There worries were well-founded. It was announced in July 2020: "New York City families will be able to keep their children home this fall and opt for a full remote school schedule regardless of medical need."[1] This was devastating as another school year would be lost to highly ineffective distance learning. Virtual teaching had been given its tryout and had failed miserably, undermining the education of children in the process.

Other states stalled reopening as well. Just after the Fourth of July in 2021, California governor Gavin Newsom ordered tougher restrictions on indoor activities for most of the state in "an attempt to slow an alarming rise of the coronavirus in nineteen counties."[2] This too had horrible consequences.

It was these mid-summer decisions that brought Rational Ground to a full rallying cry. We had let our guard down after the initial spring burst and thought that calmer heads would prevail. Instead, this was war declared on our kids!

Rational Ground would launch multiple websites and organize groups of leaders over Twitter chats to help on a local basis. We coordinated with numerous highly skilled and qualified experts in their field to testify at school boards, produce advocacy letters, and drive conversations around the true nature of lockdowns and impact on children.

Teachers' Unions Drove Science Policy for Their Own Benefit

Back in the fall of 2020, tensions were running high in anticipation of the 2020 election. President Trump decried many of the shutdowns even as his core advisors approved them time and time again. He lambasted the use of mask mandates as unnecessary and was seen frequently violating those mandates time and time again.

Leadership noticed that the impact on families and kids was undeniable. In a series of personal video messages (seemingly taken from a closet inside the CDC), Director Robert Redfield decried the impact of school closures. He noted that states were taking their school guidance way too literally. "Nothing would cause me greater sadness than to see any school district or school use our guidance as a reason not to reopen," he lamented.[3]

It was too late. Fear had taken hold. Later emails revealed that teachers' unions were instrumental in influencing guidance and keeping schools closed. This shameful act, which will no doubt have massive political repercussions, has resulted in an almost unbridgeable loss of trust between parents and teachers. This is entirely the fault of the teachers' unions.

Jeffrey Tucker, author and Team Reality member, writing for the American Institute of Economic Research, recounted a conversation with a psychologist who describes the terrible society-wide impact these decisions were having: "We see a primal fear of disease turning into mass panic. It seems almost deliberate. It is tragic. Once this starts, it could take years to repair the psychological damage."[4]

Meanwhile our health overlords kept their eye on the prize and denied any semblance of help or hope that might pull America and the world out of this anxious malaise.

PART 4

SOCIAL CONTAGION

CHAPTER 20

Your Behavior Can Stop the Virus! WRONG.

As our good friend Alex Berenson noted, "the virus is gonna virus."[1] It's nearly impossible to point to any non-pharmaceutical intervention that served to quell or stop the disease. Even drastic measures like stay-at-home orders and lockdowns seemed to exacerbate the problem as families became incubators of the disease, passing it among everyone stifled in the home with them. This was one of the biggest myths of the pandemic.

Team Apocalypse came up with an analogy asserting that all these measures taken together (lockdowns, masks, plexiglass, stay-at-home orders) would work like layers of Swiss cheese. While not foolproof, the interventions would stop the virus from transmitting. Needless to say, this analogy was full of holes.

They Are Setting Us Up for More

Of course, from a conspiratorial point of view, this very much seemed all part of a test. Larry Fink, the CEO of BlackRock (a global investment firm) and one of the advocates of the so-called Great Reset, noted in March 2022, "Behaviors are going to have to change.... You have to force behaviors."[2] Those who want to bring about a corporate-government amalgamation in order to promulgate environmental and social causes outside the democratic free market system need to control human movements to do it. To steer societal decisions without resort to democratic institutions, they *need* to control us.

The promise was if we can get everyone to do and say the right things, to wash their hands when told, then the pandemic would disappear. Then CDC director Robert Redfield said in July 2020 that we could get the pandemic totally under control if "we could get everybody to wear a mask right now."[3] Multiple studies from the CDC were published using mannequin dummies to demonstrate that mask wearing could completely stop transmission.[4] In the real world, things operate much differently. Even back in 1918 in a much more deadly epidemic, they knew that mass public directives were probably useless.

They Use Fear as a Tool

Fear, of course, is a great motivator and our health overlords used that relentlessly to get us to do their bidding. The entire wave of vaccine pronouncements was introduced again and again as a life-or-death decision. The White House in late 2021 gave a rather curious Christmastime message to the country about the status of the omicron variant: "We are intent on not letting Omicron disrupt work and school for the vaccinated. You've done the right thing, and we will get through this." Then they concluded:

> For the unvaccinated, you're looking at a winter of severe illness and death for yourselves, your families, and the hospitals you may soon overwhelm.[5]

Happy Holidays everyone, don't let that dark-robed man with the scythe inside your house. Go get jabbed, and you'll be right as rain. And if you don't, you probably deserve to die.

A large plurality of American adults did indeed get vaccinated. For the most at-risk populations the compliance was truly astounding. In some counties 99 percent of the population over sixty-five received at least one shot of the vaccination.[6] America really did bend to the will of the health overlords. The problem is that the interventions didn't stop the disease.

The effect on society has been devastating and is ongoing. Neighbors and friends saw each other as potentially fatal transmitters of the disease. Americans are now deeply distrustful of our institutions and of each other. The main cure is to realize that your behavior is your own, your decisions are your own, and both likely have very little impact on the course of the pandemic.

An aerosolized viral respiratory pathogen is not going to stop for your puny mask. It won't stop for the six feet between you. It won't stop because you're rioting for the right cause. It won't stop for a year-old newfangled vaccine. As even Team Apocalypse notes, everyone is likely to contract Covid at one point or another. How you react to this factoid could spell the trajectory of the next hundred years of this country and world.

The truth is, your behavior during the pandemic didn't change the course of much of anything as far as Covid goes. But your behavior after the pandemic might change the course of the world. You are not a vector of disease.

CHAPTER 21

Lockdowns Taught Us We Are All in This Together! WRONG.

Sadly, the economic woes and even the fall in fertility rates pale in comparison to the instant, unforeseen (or flatly ignored) health consequences caused by the lockdowns.

One of the most disgusting and damaging stats might be that 250,000 cases of child abuse went unreported.[1] Domestic abuse cases are most frequently caught by wide-eyed school administrators and teachers. This goes not only for child abuse but for domestic spousal abuse. How many bruises on a mom's face were hidden because schools required masks for drop-offs?

Mental health took a hit as well. One in four college kids had ideation of suicide in 2020. Drug use and overdoses ran rampant.[2]

Studies appear weekly confirming what almost every corner of the universe now agrees with—the lockdowns were fruitless. The authors of a review that analyzed some of the most relevant of these studies stated: "Overall, we conclude that lockdowns are not an effective way of reducing mortality rates during a pandemic."[3]

The biggest impact will be the loss in trust in our institutions. As one reader told me, "It has made me mad; it has made me sad; and I no longer trust any of our government agencies. It's also given me a lot more faith because now I know for sure that fear is a killer, but faith can get me through anything."

Lockdowns Destroyed Lives

Still others have numerous personal stories impacting their health and well-being, such as this recounting of an important female health assessment: "Two hours after I scheduled my annual mammogram I got a call back canceling it. I said I couldn't wear a mask—I'm an immune-suppressed transplant recipient. Masks are a risk for bacterial pneumonia. The hospital imaging [staff member] said I was a risk to their staff."

Another doctor chimed in about the vaccine mandates that would later plague our healthcare staffing situation:

I'm a physician who worked through the early "locked-down" days of the pandemic providing emergency anesthesia care when needed. Soon after, when "elective surgery" was restarted, surgical volume started to recover. At the end of 2020 when vaccines became available to health care workers, hospital systems started considering vaccine policies, with a game of follow the leader ensuing. One after the next implemented mandates so as not to be the only one who couldn't claim a perceived market advantage of a "fully vaccinated staff." That left no place, (or a rare place) for the unvaccinated worker to...go. Hospitals were in cahoots to leave themselves with a deepening staffing crisis, and by the end of 2021, even after providing evidence of naturally acquired immunity, and requesting medical exemptions from vaccine mandates, I was dismissed from several staff appointments—unable to practice medicine after 29 years of providing care/service to my community, with no alternative income source at the time. Good times.

The damage is done, and it is no longer theoretical.[4]

Emergency Services Were Far from Overwhelmed

Recall that the greatest fear among our health overlords was that hospitals would be overwhelmed. "Flatten the curve" described the mound-like chart produced by Gates-backed projections from the Institute for Health Metrics and Evaluation out of Washington State.[5] It was thought that a surge in cases would lead to a massive burst of hospital visits, overwhelming the systems that were positioned as the primary point of care for serious Covid illnesses and any other illnesses they would deal with on a daily basis.

Would it surprise you to learn that, compared to 2019, hospitals had *fewer* patients in 2020 and 2021? That is, in fact, the case.[6]

People Avoid Hospitals and Miss Treatments

Emergency medical services saw very low traffic as stay-at-home orders seemed to keep people from seeking treatment at ERs. That's not to say that all healthcare services were seeing fewer patients. Requests for mental health claims skyrocketed. As reported by our friend and actuary Matt Malkus, at the high point of the pandemic in March and April of 2020, mental health claims increased nearly 100 percent from the previous years for ages thirteen to eighteen while medical claims for that same age group fell 53 percent.[7] Something awful and dramatic was impacting our youth, and it would not soon abate.

One reader shared with us the story of James:

> My friend James worked for a medical device company. He
> was the guy that went into surgery to help guide surgeons
> on using their product. He was very good at what he did
> and very successful. James was married and his son and my
> son are very good friends. I coached little league football
> and baseball with James. We hunted and fished together,
> our families had dinners together. We all got together often
> to hang out on Lake Austin.
>
> James had been a college pitcher at a major D1 school,
> he was very athletic and always the life of the party—he
> was a type A personality. About a month ago I dropped
> James['s] son off at home and took my son home—they had
> been at the athletic field playing around. That night around
> 11 PM we received a call that James had taken his life with
> a shotgun in his 2 million dollar backyard. Luckily a friend
> of the family found James and not a member of his family.
> This was a complete shock. To everyone. At the funeral his
> wife said it was COVID that cause James to fall into despair.
> He was no longer allowed in hospitals to do what he did.
> He was nonessential. In his late 20s he was diagnosed with
> testicular cancer, he beat it and was in complete remission.
> But the week before he took his life he went in for a normal
> check-up to find the markers for cancer were back. They
> couldn't locate cancer anywhere but the signs were there.
> He was vaccinated. Did the vaccine cause his cancer to come
> back? I hope we find out one day.

These assaults on life, liberty, and the pursuit of happiness must
not go unpunished. The fear driven by the pandemic might be the

single biggest killer in all of this. During the late summer 2020, I received this message from a Rational Ground follower:

> Justin, BOTH of my elderly parents died this year, four months apart, Dad from undiagnosed glioblastoma in June, and Mom from undiagnosed artery blockage causing [a] stroke last week. Four months apart. They locked down and were afraid to go out at all, even for medical care. Our family is devastated and will never be the same. Tragic!!

(I provide dozens of other testimonials—some amusing, many heartbreaking—in appendix 2 of this book.)

Fear kills. Lockdowns are devastating. As noted by many experts, the total impact of the lockdowns won't be known for some time. By all accounts the number of deaths from lockdown impacts will far exceed those of the disease itself.

CHAPTER 22

The Pandemic Led to Lots of Sex and a Baby Boom! WRONG.

Consider two star-crossed lovers in San Francisco. After an evening of drinking turned into a one-night stand, the slightly embarrassed couple wakes to find a set of health inspectors at their door.

"I'm sorry, but you cannot leave this apartment," says an inspector. "According to city guidelines if you have had intimate relations with someone not of your household you must quarantine for fourteen days."

A one-night stand turns into a fortnight plod with people who barely know one another. Talk about a buzz killer.

This might sound like fiction, but for a stretch of time in late 2020, those were the rules in San Francisco. You could date, but if you kissed, you were required to quarantine. Together. Local news outlets and opinion pieces buoyed this notion.

Dating was dangerous, and probably morally wrong. As local radio station KQED put it, "Let's get this straight: during the COVID-19 pandemic, there is no 'safe way' to have sex with someone you don't live and quarantine with." Experts consulted recommended "wearing a mask" and "choosing positions that minimize face-to-face contact." They also recommend that you "keep it quick."[1]

At this point, logic and reason had left the city limits.[2]

Love in the Time of Covid Gets Very Weird

Across the country in New York City, health officials were under no illusion that a scary bug like Covid would keep people from getting funky. The Covid Sex Guidance download gives assurances:

"People who are fully vaccinated (at least two weeks have passed since they got a single-dose vaccine or the second dose of a two-dose vaccine) can more safely go on dates, make out and have sex."

The guide continues: "Before you hook up . . ." ask a bunch of ridiculous questions of your make-out partner like if they've been tested and if they've been recently exposed. In the section "Play safer," they have some keep recommendations, namely: "Avoid sex parties and large gatherings. If you do attend, follow COVID-19 precautions." They suggest you "Enjoy sex virtually . . . sexy Zoom parties." Most importantly: "Wear a face mask, even during sex!" They suggest you should "make it kinky . . . be creative with sexual positions and physical barriers that allow sexual contact while preventing close face-to-face contact." They end with the vital advice: "Wash hands and sex toys with soap and warm water. Disinfect keyboards and touch screens you share with others."[3]

It turns out every single major city put out its own advice on having sex during the pandemic, and the way these were phrased says more about the inner workings of blue city employees' imaginations than it does about how the actual act is accomplished. The city of Washington, D.C., suggested you wait on sex if either of you aren't feeling up to par: "Sex and close contact will be waiting for you when you are feeling better."[4] The city of Austin tried to keep it weird. Their advice: "Just because you have to stay physically distant from your honey, doesn't mean you can't go on a great date! . . . Go on a narrated walk-talk on the phone while walking around your neighborhood. Describe what you see around you to your partner (ex. flowers, trees, houses, general things that you are attracted to and why)."[5] The American Sexual Health Association declared: "You are your safest sex partner," and "Consider taking a break from in-person dates."[6]

In short, all of the experts agreed: basically, you shouldn't be dating or having sex with anyone during Covid, and you *really* shouldn't be exchanging those nasty, infectious fluids and droplets.

Population Collapse Likely Accelerates

The jury is out on what impact lockdowns and the pandemic have on our population, but it can't be good. While popular opinion has it that the world is overpopulated, the truth of the matter is that much of the Western world is depopulating faster than you can say *infertility*.

In the bestselling 2006 book *America Alone*, Mark Steyn notes that the incredible falling birth rates across the world mean that you can *either* choose lavish social spending programs *or* no kids—but not both. As he quips, without children, there won't be any kids to stick the bill with.[7]

Along with terrible employment impacts, there are equally concerning birth numbers coming out of government agencies. It's not a pretty sight. Typically, we expect over 350,000 births every month in the United States. If we fall below those numbers, then we can't replace the population that dies each month.

The average number of live births across the country dropped from 311,833 births in January 2020 to 298,583 births in January 2021.

There are 167 million women in the United States, and so the birth rate bottoms out at 1.7 births per female. The inexorable fact is that you need about 2.1 births to keep up with ongoing deaths just to replace the population. Many countries in Europe are at the lowest low of 1.3 births per woman—from which no society has ever returned in history.[8]

Obviously, the uncertainty of lockdowns is having a dramatic impact on births. If we look at just one state, my home of California, we can see the impact that the lockdowns had. Births in February in 2021 fell to 30,080 from 34,019 in 2019. And this is an even bigger decline from 37,866 in 2016. 2021: 30,080. In other words, over the course of five years the number of births in the month of February dropped nearly 20 percent.[9]

Some thought the stay-at-home orders would wind up bringing more whoopie into our lives. They were wrong.

More ominously, if we look at Google search trends for the word "infertility" over the last five years, we get some interesting results. The pandemic, the pandemic response, and maybe something else are *not* helping with childbearing. The data shows a threefold increase in the number of searches for the word "infertility" starting in early 2021.[10]

CHAPTER 23

During Covid, All Lives Matter! WRONG.

T he entire nation, it seemed, was walking on eggshells—and who could blame the lay citizens for succumbing to that nervousness? They turn on the news to witness physical altercations on planes over masking. They hear about their neighbors getting kicked out of a supermarket or yelled at for not donning the mask properly. They see the latest captured phone video of, for instance, a brave paddle-boarder being chased down the beach by a squad of police officers—or watch a host of skater kids removed from a skate park and looking on in shock as the police fill it with sand.

Later, children and teens were turned away from museums because they didn't have their biomedical identifications with them. (Never mind that they couldn't legally get a vaccination—they just wouldn't be able to enjoy life until they got the jab). And of course, tens of thousands of people lost their jobs because they wouldn't get vaccinated.

The same OSHA confab that turned a blind eye to the ridiculousness of mask mandates was all too eager to throw itself into the vaccine mandate scene and declare that Covid was a toxic substance to be regulated in the workplace. The Biden administration saw to it that federal mandates flew far and wide. In the end, most did not pass legal muster. But the damage and fearmongering were replete across government.

The BLM Riots Blessed by the CDC

There was one moment during the pandemic that suspended all impositions of social distancing, masks, and fear of Covid—the summer protests of 2020. But you had to be at the *right* kind of protest. Or rather the Left. If you were protesting the lockdowns, that was a no-go. But a Black Lives Matter march received all kinds of special exemptions.

Don't get me wrong. Those protestors have every right to their opinions, as did the numerous lockdown protesters, but the contrast in reaction from lay pundits to science experts led to innumerable moments of hypocrisy. Epidemiologists and virologists who days before had warned against crowds gathering in one place now suddenly changed their tune and declared that the purpose of the protests was just too important to worry about Covid in the face of the subject matter at hand.

Jennifer Nuzzo, a Johns Hopkins epidemiologist, tweeted, "We should always evaluate the risks and benefits of efforts to control the virus. In this moment the public health risks of not protesting to demand an end to systematic racism greatly exceed the harm of the virus."[1]

NBC News took the cake with a pair of tweets just an hour apart on June 14, 2020. One headline reads: "Rally for Black Trans Lives Draws Packed Crowd to Brooklyn Museum Plaza." An hour later they lamented: "President Trump plans to rally his supporters next Saturday for the first time.... But health experts are questioning that decision."[2]

When protests erupted against lockdowns, the state of California intervened to thwart any lawsuit from progressing. The state argued: "Because there is no vaccine or even widely effective treatment against COVID-19, state public health officials have determined that mass gatherings present an unacceptable danger of spreading the virus."

Think the same should apply to BLM protests and riots? Think again. Just a month or two later when BLM protests grew violent, authorities had almost moved in to quell the damage when Governor Gavin Newsom tweeted: "Protesters have the right to protest peacefully—not be harassed."[3]

The Florida "Angel of Death"—Was a Virtue Signaling Hypocrite

Daniel Uhlfeder, a Florida lawyer, would infamously dress up as the grim reaper and appear on Florida beaches that Governor DeSantis had reopened shortly after the first lockdowns. His statement was clear: if you don't stay home, you are reaping death. A month or two later, Daniel could be seen at a BLM rally with hundreds of protestors out of costume and unmasked.

Don Lemon of CNN, witnessing the mass of lockdown protests building across the country, is seen with a then employed Chris Cuomo. Both of them are dismayed at the crowds, and Lemon yells into the camera, "Who the hell do you think you are?...Stay at home!"[4]

A month later he had changed his tune. Lemon lauded the massive crowds at BLM "peaceful protests." Nancy Pelosi was disgusted by the beleaguered Americans outside protesting the quashing of their jobs, but weeks later her heart was "warmed" by the BLM protests in full force.[5]

With all of this physical violence, confrontation, and contrasting hypocrisy, one perhaps should not fault the lay citizen and his desire to mask up constantly, dutifully accept the jab, publicly acknowledge the glorious lockdowns, and change all of his social media avatars to a mask-mummified version of himself adorned with syringes and BLM stickers showing his compliance.

CHAPTER 24

"Covid Karens" Really Have Everyone's Best Interest at Heart! WRONG.

So much of public, grueling ostracism stemmed from these three measures: masks, lockdowns, and mandates. They became the holy triad of non-pharmaceutical interventions (NPIs). It created massive strains on families, colleagues, neighbors, and educators, and every industry felt the pressure to comply.

Denying the efficacy or throwing the slightest shade on the mandate of vaccines was not just public anathema—it could end your career in an instant and disabuse you of any presence on the interwebs. Fostering obedience to these measures was easy. The mechanism of virtue signaling created its own enforcement mechanism.

The Karens.

The term "Karen" was coined to refer to an individual who exuded great anxiety around the enforcement of regulations. Many of the Rational Ground readers took these encounters in stride and tried their best to have some fun with the situation.[1]

Love Degenerates into Neurosis

It's one thing to hold a phobia of other people; it's quite another to look at your loved ones and brand them as vectors of disease. One college lad made his way back home via plane to his parents for the holiday season 2020. His family picked him up, requested that he remain masked from the moment he got off the plane, and plopped him into the back of their car, which had been makeshift retrofitted into a level-three biohazard lab. Mom and Dad had outfitted the back of the seat with ceiling-to-floor plastic sheeting two-layers thick. The college son does a TikTok of the scene and notes, "My fam decided to pimp out the welcoming car."[2]

Before you conclude that this was a rare moment, we have it on good authority from virologists and epidemiologists that this might be considered good practice by our health overlords. Andy Slavitt, a senior advisor to the White House on coronavirus, noted that he was going to quarantine his son in his garage when he came home for a visit. "Then there's the matter of college kids. We have one. I love him. So, I mean this with no disrespect: stay away from them. Keep them from the people you love. Shun them if they come home for Thanksgiving. Have them sleep in the garage. Have them wear masks."[3]

Later, Slavitt would delete the tweet and claim he was joking, but the context and rapport of the tweet seemed entirely authentic and in-character for him.[4]

This same gambit was employed for the next holiday season as well. Psychologist Lisa Tamour told *CBS Mornings* that, if you intend to have family over for Thanksgiving, why not mix it up a bit and cater to those untimely fears? "If it feels like it's going to be weird, maybe make it kind of fun," Tamour told the hosts, "say 'We're going to start with hors d'oeuvres in the garage, you know, we'll have drinks, we'll do our rapid tests, and then come on in,' right?"[5]

CHAPTER 25

You Must Keep Sacrificing to Quell the Disease! WRONG.

The irony behind the world's first murder is that philosophers have inferred an axiom from Cain's rebuke to God, "Am I my brother's keeper?" The inference is an inversion of that guilty cry: "You *are indeed* your brother's keeper." This aligns nicely with the admonition of Jesus Christ who conveyed the couplet: "Thou shalt love the Lord thy God with all thy heart, and with all thy soul, and with all thy mind. This is the first and great commandment. And the second is like unto it, Thou shalt love thy neighbor as thyself." (Matthew 22:37–39). Worship and charity are two of the pillars of the Christian creed.

There is of course no Constitutional requirement for you to love your neighbor, and the government may not enjoin you to worship in any specific way (or forbid you to worship, more accurately). There is, however, an American tradition of service and community that might even be termed a societal norm or expectation. As Alexis de Tocqueville put it, canvassing America in the nineteenth century, "I must say that I have often seen Americans make great and real sacrifices to the public welfare; and have noticed a hundred instances in which they hardly ever failed to lend faithful support to one another."[1] The American altruist emboldens our society, and that selfsame spirit can indeed be found across the world in many cultures.

Enter the pandemic.

Doing What the Government Says Is Not the Same as Doing Right

We might ask: What is our obligation to our fellow man amid a viral respiratory pathogenic episode? What kind of sacrifice should we expect from others to quell the disease that threatens us and our families?

These are certainly worthy questions, but they are not the questions at hand. They do not frame the situation we are experiencing but exist in a world where there is no greed, corruption, or closet tyrant trying to take advantage of our good will. We should instead ask, what is the role of the government in compelling sacrifice to stop a virus? What kind of rights do we have in the face of such force?

Altruism is not a government program. Compelled sacrifice is a very real possibility when the people have granted authority to a representative government, but there is no duty-bound obligation to adhere to proposed mandates. You must, of course, suffer the consequences where a legal authority has the means to conjure violence and force compliance—but you cannot force a man into altruism, especially when that man believes that the actions you are trying to compel don't actually help at all, or that they are harmful.

Applying this to our COVID-19 policies, the stay-at-home orders were indeed a great sacrifice for many, many families. If you failed to follow those mandates you could be detained, arrested, fined, and imprisoned. On the other hand, it is perfectly reasonable for one to feel a sense of pride in performing an offering that you believe will help others. Authentic belief is the separating motive between compelled behavior and a willing sacrifice. Altruism can only be had with a trust that one's actions will indeed make a positive difference. You cannot legislate morality as the saying goes.

The problem is that there is almost zero evidence that *any* of the COVID-19 mandates had *any* positive effect on the outcome of the pandemic. After the examination of four hundred studies, the Brownstone Institute concludes, "Nearly all governments have attempted compulsory measures to control the virus, but no government can claim success. The research indicates that mask mandates, lockdowns, and school closures have had no discernible impact of virus trajectories."[2]

Nothing the Government Forced on Us Worked

Social distancing, lockdowns, stay-at-home orders, masking, and quarantines: all of these had no measurable effect on the course of the pandemic. An obligation to sacrifice one's freedoms, wealth, time, happiness, ease, and comforts to stop a disease can only hold efficacy when there is proof that the sacrifice works. We don't call it love when a mother cat licks her kitten to death. We call it obsession.

After the 1918 pandemic, one doctor writing in a Des Moines newspaper opined: "The people are perfectly willing to do whatever needs to be done. But they dislike greatly the inconvenience to themselves only to learn later that what they did was not necessary."[3]

The lockdowns, which picked specific industry winners and losers in the 2020 economy, deeply infringed on the core tenets of our right as Americans to the pursuit of happiness. The lack of reason or logic amplified the frustration that many felt throughout the pandemic. In New York City, a bar could remain open if it served the right type of food. In London you could travel openly if you could demonstrate that your business provided substantial financial benefit to the country.

The Institutions Failed and Keep Failing

For masks, the incredible mesh of confusion and ridiculous policies greatly degraded one's trust in any other interventions. You must wear your mask on your way to a table, but you can take it off to eat. Your preschool child must don the mask for most of the school day but must remove it to take a midday nap lying next to the other children. The chaos ran deep in every walk of life and sometimes differed per county. One restaurant in Los Angeles County was barred from hosting dine-in hosts, whereas a restaurant five hundred feet away in Orange County welcomed maskless diners all day long. Common sense was nowhere to be found, and its absence inhibited any sense that the measures taken were for the "greater good."

The governor of Florida, Ron DeSantis, whose actions during the pandemic stood out in sharp contrast to those of almost every other governor in the country, implemented legislation that put specific triggers in place to ensure that no county health director could declare an emergency with unending powers.[4] The county must prove with data-driven analysis that there was truly a need for compelled action on the citizenry in reaction to a health crisis. For most of the pandemic, a simple roll call of cases rising was enough to shut down entire school systems and businesses with only hours' notice. Unlike most every other legislative or executive initiative, there was no specific justification needed to implement these. In many cases, color tiers and trigger levels were set by the state or the county to automatically implement some type of intervention. These proved to be unwieldy and moved like a goal post on wheels.

In the end, government could compel you to action, but it could not truly claim that action as a willing sacrifice. If there is no native, authentic drive behind a requirement for self-sacrifice, the bill eventually comes due, usually in the form of degraded trust, electoral retribution, or worse, violence.

CHAPTER 26

Covid Is like Nothing We've Ever Seen Before! WRONG.

Covid is a challenging infection, but in the panoply of diseases, the fear of the disease was worse than the disease itself. We were in a battle, the authorities claimed—a war even—comparable to some of the greatest disasters in history. Yet curiously, those same authorities have not actually learned from history itself.

All of this has happened before.

Federal lockdowns empowered state behemoths with a massive surge of wealth to create an army of health directors and contact tracers. These health bureaucrats went on to issue massively stringent "recommendations" for their "constituents." California, supposedly the apex of American culture and sophistication, saw some of the most draconian and ridiculous measures employed to curb the pandemic.

Examples abound. In May 2020, to impede those hooligans in Venice Beach, the local government filled in the world-famous skateboard park and pavilion with sand. In Huntington Beach, California, at the height of the mandatory, state-wide stay-at-home order, news choppers showed police officers chasing down a lone paddleboarder just offshore. Multiple units are dispatched to arrest him. There were many other egregious instances of such lunacy.[1]

Nasty Authoritarians Arose during the Italian Black Plague

Yet, as the Good Book says, there is nothing new under the sun. For example, the nineteenth-century Italian author Alessandro Manzoni poured over hundreds of seventeenth-century journals while writing his acclaimed novel, *The Betrothed*. This work follows a pair of lovers clamoring to get married in the middle of the plague which hit Milan in 1630. Manzoni recounts the chaos of seventeenth-century Italy as a very *real* deadly virus struck the heart of the civilized world. Manzoni could have been writing about the pandemic-spun chaos in 2020. Four hundred years later, we don't seem to have learned a thing.

Manzoni recounts a massive wave of rumors of "unclean people" spreading the plague: "The city, already tumultuously inclined, was now turned upside down," he writes. To stave off infection they started to burn and destroy everything that might be infected. "Owners of the houses, with lighted straw, burned the besmeared spots; and passers-by stopped, gazed, shuddered, murmured." Suspicions rose. "Strangers, suspected of this alone, and at that time easily recognized by their dress, were arrested by the people in the streets, and consigned to prison. Here interrogations and examinations were made of captured, captors, and witnesses."[2]

Further rumors took hold, claiming these forces would use tainted oil and water for "anointing" walls and benches. If you didn't follow things to an exacting degree, measures were taken against you. "In the church of Sant' Antonio, on the day of I know not what solemnity, an old man, more than eighty years of age, was observed, after kneeling in prayer, to sit down, first, however, dusting the bench with his cloak. 'That old man is anointing the benches!' exclaimed with one voice some women, who witnessed the act."

> The people...fell upon the old man; they tore his gray locks, heaped upon him blows and kicks, and dragged him out half dead, to convey him to prison, to the judges, to torture....I think he could not have survived many moments.

A group called the *Monatti* came to power—unelected officials appointed to "enforce good government" (not unlike county health directors)—these "exercised all kinds of tyranny" over the citizenry. "The strictest orders were laid upon these people; the severest penalties threatened to them; stations were assigned them; and commissaries...placed over them:...magistrates and nobles were appointed in every district, with authority to enforce good government summarily."[3]

We're Repeating a Shameful History, and We Don't Even Realize It

Nearly four hundred years later and a continent away, numerous companies came into being to "shepherd" restaurants through the onerous tasks of meeting Los Angeles County health department guidelines. The going price was several thousand dollars of what amounted to protection money. Magically, health directors would then sign off and give permission for your little enterprise to operate.[4]

Eventually, almost one-third of all restaurants in California would go out of business.[5]

Back in Manzoni's seventeenth-century Italy,

> They entered the houses like masters, like enemies; and, not to mention their plunder, and how they treated the unhappy

creatures reduced by the plague to pass through such hands, they laid them—these infected and guilty hands—on the healthy—children, parents, husbands, wives, threatening to drag them to the Lazzaretto, unless they redeemed themselves, or were redeemed, with money. At other times they set a price upon their services, refusing to carry away bodies already corrupted, for less than so many *scudi*.[6]

The Lazzaretto was the quarantine house. In our pandemic, major university campuses designated specific dorms for the Covid-positive students to be sequestered. My own stepdaughter away at college could guess the spread of Covid on campus based on how many lights would show up in the quarantine tower each evening.

In Australia, the government proudly constructed and utilized the internment-style camps for positive cases hoping to pursue a zero-Covid policy for the entire continent. As of this writing, cases are up *thirteen thousand percent* from the time they declared their umpteenth lockdown.[7]

Surely the seventeenth-century Italian restrictions were lifted and the dictatorial enforcers disbanded? Not so fast, says Manzoni, "Such a state of things went on and took effect up to a certain period; but, with the increase of deaths and desolation, and the terror of the survivors, these officers came to be, as it were, exempted from all supervision; they constituted themselves, the *monatti* especially, arbiters of everything."[8]

"The arbiters of everything."

"Exempt from all supervision."

PART 5

GOVERNMENT POWERGRABS

CHAPTER 27

The Rollout of Vaccines Was Bumpy but Fair! WRONG.

I n the 2011 film *Contagion*, a global virus with massive transmission rates and high mortality rates was unleashed across the world. Due to the limited supply of the vaccine, a lottery was determined based on your birthday—a seemingly fair process avoiding even the appearance of politics.

Not so with the rollout of COVID-19 vaccines. With limited supply of the vaccine in demand at the end of 2021, it was determined that a pecking order be devised based primarily on necessity. In other words many states chose to forego age as a primary decision mechanism and use "essential jobs" as the criteria for rollout. The CDC relied on a young millennial wunderkind apparently to draw up its prioritization plan.

The plan called for phases and tiers of vaccine rollouts to healthcare workers and teachers at the front of the line. Age was a secondary consideration.[1] Health organizations tried to stem demand from those at risk clamoring for the vaccine. New York governor Andrew Cuomo threatened steep fines for practitioners who tried to administer the vaccine outside of the pecking order the federal institutions had implemented.[2]

This proved to be a fiasco. Within days both Florida and Texas governors decided against the CDC recommendations and reorganized prioritization with age and health risk as the vital determinants.[3] It was clear from the get-go that the CDC had erred (again) in this recommendation, which was based primarily on interest groups and not on science. By January, the CDC adopted the age and risk-first recommendation for distribution of the vaccine that any reasonable grownup would have put in place from the start.[4]

CHAPTER 28

Government Scientists Are Doing Okay, Considering the Challenge! WRONG.

Let's not fool ourselves. Most of the American mainstream media would gladly weld you inside your apartment if given the chance. The same can be said for our virologist class of epidemiologists. The infectious disease community was intent on saving the world—even if it meant burning the world down to accomplish it. They viewed themselves as Dustin Hoffman from the movie *Outbreak*, heroically trying to chase down and isolate the source of a deadly contagion. In truth, their actions played out like a scene from *Ghostbusters* when dopey EPA inspector Walter Peck (played by William Atherton) shuts down the control grid and lets loose a ghostly chaos on the city.

Videos from China Were Cherry-Picked by Media for Gruesome Effect

Flashback to late 2019, when videos began to surface from China showing random people being felled by some unseen force. At work, on the subway, on the street—the videos were disturbing to say the least. In some cases, the videos were explicitly linked to the outbreak of a new viral respiratory pathogen. In other cases, it was unclear if there was any connection at all. The ambiguity fed the imaginations of writers and editors everywhere.[1]

More video began to surface of contagion-uniform–clad workers hustling dead bodies away, or, worse yet, officials welding entire families into their apartments with wedged locks. "Two videos show all floors of a residential building in Jiangsu-China were blocked by welding fence because a confirmed case was found in it," read one tweet from the region in late January 2020.[2]

A video in February would show the aftermath when officials later pried open the bolts on the apartment of one unfortunate set of forced homebodies who were dead inside—presumably deceased from this invisible menace that was definitely coming to a city near you. The tenor of the mitigation measures went from "wash your hands" to "weld them inside" within two weeks.

"These extreme limitations on population movement have been quite successful," said notorious lockdown proponent Michael Osterholm in *Nature* magazine in March 2020.[3] The World Health Organization (WHO) lauded praise on the China in their February 2020 report: "China's uncompromising and rigorous use of non-pharmaceutical measures to contain transmission of the COVID-19 virus in multiple settings provides vital lessons for the global response."[4]

The World Health Organization Belongs Lock, Stock, and Barrel to China

The WHO is designed to act as the gatekeeper for these type of outbreaks, but China hid their disaster until it was too late. It's clear from satellite photos that something in China was afoot as early as August 2019. Photos show heightened activity at hospitals and research facilities in and around Wuhan.[5] The WHO in early 2020 famously denied there was any chance of human-to-human Covid transmission—essentially parroting what their Chinese counterparts lied to them about.[6] The Lunar year was afoot, and many Chinese were traveling in celebration. Those travel destinations would quickly become a hotbed of activity for Covid. This too answers the question around why Italy fared so poorly: over the past decade, while Italy's birthrate continued to plummet, a strong economic tie was made with China to help with the labor shortage around the production of leather goods in Italy.[7]

The epitome of the WHO kowtowing to Chinese authorities was when Bruce Aylward, a Canadian epidemiologist and senior advisor to the WHO, gave an interview to a news agency in Taiwan in early 2020. When asked why the WHO excluded Taiwan from official membership in the WHO, Aylward went silent, exclaiming he couldn't hear the question. The interviewer asked several times. Aylward then disconnected altogether. China holds immense sway over WHO appointments and activities.[8]

The WHO director general, Dr. Tedros Adhanom Ghebreyesus, exclaimed that Chinese efforts were "beyond words," adding, "so is China's commitment to transparency and to supporting other countries."[9] In fact, the Chinese approach was disastrous, and the cover-up was borderline criminal. The litany of lies and delay along with misreporting from agencies charged with disseminating the truth caused a significant worldwide lag in preparing for the ultimate outbreak.

The Trump administration would subsequently pull out of the WHO in protest of the utter failure of the organization. "I must say the reason we left the World Health Organization was because we came to believe that it was corrupt," Secretary of State Mike Pompeo said. "It had been politicized. It was bending a knee to General Secretary Xi Jinping in China. I hope that's not the case here with what they've announced today."[10]

CHAPTER 29

The Pandemic Brings Out the Best in Our Leaders! WRONG.

In August 2020, as the second wave of Covid began to hit across the country, attendees of MTV's Video Music Awards were granted exemptions from New York City's extreme pandemic rules, requiring out-of-state visitors to quarantine themselves for fourteen days upon arrival or face massive fines. Not so these celebrities.[1]

The next month, Speaker of the House Nancy Pelosi, who verbally championed business shutdowns as a means to stop the pandemic, was caught getting her hair styled by a hairdresser who was otherwise forbidden to take clients in San Francisco.[2]

And then there was the Dinner Heard Round the World. It took place in November 2020 in the Napa Valley of California as Governor Gavin Newsom ate and cavorted at The French Laundry, one of the finest (and most expensive) restaurants in the world. Photos showed Newsom maskless, sitting with people who were *not* part of his household.[3] The hypocrisy stunned even his most ardent supporters. Across the whole nation, the hypocrisy of government officials was astounding.[4]

A modern-day Manzoni would not be surprised. He may as well have been writing about *us* from his perch in the nineteenth century.

Government Hypocrisy Is Nothing New

Team Apocalypse would frequently use clippings from the 1918 Spanish flu pandemic to justify mask mandates and other enforcement mechanisms as a popular precedent for today's Covid response. A *San Francisco Chronicle* front page headline from October 25 of that same year read in all caps: "WEAR YOUR MASK! COMMANDS DRASTIC NEW ORDINANCE." Seen below the headline were five masked faces of various leaders of the city. Over the course of the 1918 pandemic, three thousand arrests and fines would be made for mask mandate infringements in California alone.[5]

What's less well known was that there was a substantial reaction to the extremist ways of local governments even back then.[6]

The proto-Karens were along for the ride during the Spanish flu as well. We know now that the masks in 1918 did little to stop the spread (if anything), yet you can practically hear San Francisco mayor London Breed through these words of John A. Britton in a letter printed in the October 25, 1918, *San Francisco Chronicle*: "A week ago I laughed at the idea of the mask," Britton wrote, "I wanted to be independent. I did not realize that the cost of such independence was the lives of others. Today I bow my head and wish I had the military authority to make every one in San Francisco wear a mask, so that the Influenza would be stamped out here as quickly as at Mare island, where that authority was present."[7]

Hypocrisy was common then as now.[8] And what did it all signify? Fast-forward to 1920. *The Spokesman-Review* of February 11 notes:

"At the end of the first wave there was a general agreement that the measure had proved ineffective."

The writer goes on to blame people in part for not wearing the mask consistently and says that if the *right* mask were worn *properly* it *might* have worked, but "this is not enough to warrant the compulsory use of masks by all the population."[9]

Much of the "science" from 1918 to 1920 was equally impressive as that of our present-day government science gurus. A widely circulated report in the 1920s claimed influenza was passed from the doffing of hats. "During the devastating epidemic of flu, the Turks in Europe escaped because," it was supposed, "they never removed their turbans." Also "in support of this contention, it was pointed out that the great majority of victims were of the male sex. A traveler found influenza to be unusually severe in Mexico, where, as he remarked, there is so much hat-doffing."[10]

It doesn't take a flu outbreak to bring out the government propaganda. An economic slowdown or war will do. During the 1930s and 1940s, the Works Progress Administration subsidized an entire army of artists and writers to push authoritarian healthcare propaganda. Labor and the creation of jobs was the focus, but the program also recruited artists who created thousands of posters touting local theater and warning against tuberculosis and disease spreading in inadequate public housing.[11]

Tech Giants Were in Bed with Government Charlatans

The propaganda of our own day with Covid is well-established. Tech companies came out in force to help push government policies. The ever-present redesigned Google logo was chief among them. One Google logo depicted all the letters of the iconic tech company, fully masked and the last getting ready to distribute the vaccine to his other alphabetic friends.

In Santa Monica, California, the city devised a hotline for people to call if they found infringements. One online advertisement and social media post declared: "Remember, you can report issues with face mask compliance to 3-1-1, and a Health Ambassador will do a business check."[12]

CHAPTER 30

Government Action Saved the Economy! WRONG.

The first sign that something was amiss (and perhaps ominously so) was in March 2020 when a run on toilet paper began in the days leading up the federal two-week shutdown. My wife and I high-tailed it to Costco to get one of their infamous thirty-roll Kirkland slabs to haul home. When we got there the line had already formed snakelike around the building and through the parking lot. Like anything at Costco, it was fairly organized and linear, sending us on a direct path to the back rooms, guided by dozens of workers throughout the building giving a constant reminder to "only take one package." That was the beginning of the supply chain problems that persist even at the time of the writing of this book.

The paucity of TP in those weeks became a running joke, but the empty aisles spread like their own virus to other sections of the store: yogurt, ramen, flour, sugar, all with signs limiting customers to one purchased item. This wasn't just about demand—in many ways it was about shifting demands. We were expected to expect less, and to like it. Or at least to take what we could when we could and shut up the rest of the time.[1]

That's just one industry. Imagine that scene playing out in every pillar of the economy all at once. In some places, the effect was one not merely of inconvenience but of guilt, sorrow, and spiritual turmoil.

Take the sad work of death. Workers in hospice facilities had to develop instructional materials to teach families how to use FaceTime, Zoom, Microsoft Teams, and other video conference tools so they could say goodbye to their dying loved one because they were not allowed in facilities. As one worker told me: "Those families will never recover from that trauma."

Things Were Good as 2020 Dawned

For many businesses, 2020 began with great optimism. Then the signs of something amiss started to come in.

One colleague told me, "We got the call first from one of my daughters' schools talking about an extended spring break (fourteen days to flatten the curve), then our former governor declared some of us nonessential. My wife goes to Costco and is scared to death by a person in a gas mask.... Then the city parks decide the virus is like nuclear fallout and put up caution tape around all the playgrounds. My other daughter with Down syndrome lost access to months of needed therapies and friends, my business development went from optimism to not hearing from a customer for ten months. Small businesses were often hit the hardest."

Effects resonated through society as the economy was brought to a screeching halt.[2]

The impact went far beyond the economic. People's lives were affected in unfathomable, detrimental ways.[3] Many parents had to deal with a flurry of needs from their children that they had never before encountered. Tech support was quickly added to the skill set required to ensure any kind of distance learning experience for their kids. Routines were needlessly upended.[4]

I remember distinctly the anger I felt towards Governor Newsom in California when we went to the park and found the authorities had padlocked the swings. My daughters were despondent. It seems that many parents encountered these same frustrations, made worse by occasional run-ins with officious citizens in retail stores and even outside—the least likely location to actually get Covid.

One mother described to me how she tried to sneak her kids onto a playground without masks in the spring of 2021. A dutiful Karen had put herself on patrol there. She burst out of her car and started yelling at the mom and kids to put their masks on. Clearly, a good number of citizens felt duty-bound to enforce these capricious rules of their own accord. It's amazing what kind of self-aggrandizing virtue signaling was enjoyed by many folks during the pandemic. When the government shuts down your day job, pays you to stay home, claims death as the outcome for any human interaction, and broadcasts that day and night, wars can start between previously peaceable neighbors.

Chaos Reigns When Economies Collapse

When you stop the wheel of the world from moving, chaos ensues. To compensate for lockdown disruptions to families and businesses, the government, under the direction of President Trump, Vice President Mike Pence, Treasury Secretary Steven Mnuchin, and the Covid task force ramped up an unprecedented campaign compensating companies for retaining full-time employees and allowing for interest-free loans to help them through the hardships. Then the government locked their plows in the field, paid them for the inconvenience, and asked them to sit at home awaiting further instructions.

The administration of remittances and loans was divvied out to the Small Business Administration and the Department of the Treasury. Within weeks, a trillion dollars was out the door to buoy up the economy.

It will take years, if not decades, to show the final impact on the world economy, but the initial results were not terribly impressive. In July 2020, Yelp indicated that more than half of U.S. business closures in its virtual yellow pages were permanent.[5]

By August, Bloomberg.com was raising the red flag that small businesses were dying by the thousands. They deemed it a "wave of silent failures."[6]

Meanwhile businesses such as Amazon, Walmart, Zoom, and various delivery services saw their biggest revenue gains ever.

Of course, along the way the strangest government stratagems were being employed to keep people on payrolls and simultaneously pay them not to work. By the end of July nearly three in ten young people were neither working nor learning. Some economists refer to this as the "disconnection rate." The direct connection to Covid policies was the culprit.[7]

By the end of 2021, the tension between state handouts, federal government advances, and a massive wave of open job positions had everyone bewildered. There were so many people out of work, yet a huge number of jobs were going unfilled.

Reopening Went FUBAR Due to Idiotic Planning

The reopening of the economy proved an even more embarrassing endeavor for the powers that be. Many states proposed "phases" to show who could go about their business. In New York Phase 3 (Summer 2020), it was determined that the following businesses could get back to work:

- Dog runs
- Tattoo parlors
- Spas, including massage parlors
- Personal care salons (hair salons reopened in Phase 2, but Phase 3 will see the reopening of nail salons, tanning salons)
- The Parks Department is reopening basketball, handball, tennis, bocce and volleyball courts[8]

Due to the increase in Covid cases, Governor Gavin Newsom ordered certain industries and businesses in nineteen counties in California to scale down their operations. Fresno, Kern, Kings, Merced, and Tulare in the Central Valley were among the counties affected. However, the governor's own winery stayed open despite all the closures.[9] The hypocrisy was palpable.

Major corporations such as McDonald's slowed and stalled their reopening plans. Restaurants suffered massive losses, and many have yet to recover fully even in 2022. Twenty-one states paused their reopening efforts altogether, following the lead of strict lockdown locales such as New York City and San Francisco. Massive closures occurred among high-trafficked businesses such as bars and gyms. Elective surgeries were halted. Well into 2022 masks are still required at many of these establishments and sometimes everywhere in entire locales.

CHAPTER 31

The Worst Is Over and Things Are Returning to Normal! WRONG.

As of this writing, COVID-19 is picking up again in Asian countries. At the beginning of 2022, numerous news outlets had lauded the successful measures employed by China to quell the disease. Since the fateful start of the pandemic in late 2019, China has been not only the initial source of the virus but, frankly, the source of all viral misinformation. Its lockdowns were adopted by regimes across the world with disastrous results.

China Is Swallowing Its Own Poison

China has put Shanghai on lockdown in anticipation of a massive wave of Covid cases. Videos making their way out of the city show massive arrests of people violating Covid curfew. One video shows a man violently beaten to the ground as authorities attempt to restrain him. Another video shows a woman attempting to flee "volunteers" dressed in full bio gear as they push her up against a pole and repeatedly hit her.[1] I don't speak Mandarin, but I suppose they are yelling at her, "I'm doing this for your health!"

Food became a scarcity as rationing and delivery of goods was centralized. One Twitter user described how one person in each building is designated to go to the lobby to retrieve rations for that day. The designee is given full PPE garb and has a limited time frame in which to grab the rations and distribute it to various apartments.

More video from Shanghai shows multiple individuals being pulled out of a small crowd by these same ever-present officials and carted off to various vans waiting behind a fence. One fellow tries to resist and is shoved straight up against the fencing. Half a dozen women fall to their knees and abase themselves before the volunteers (as they are known), pleading not to be taken away. Panic has set in.[2]

It was thought that the initial videos released out of China may have been propaganda tactics to send fear across the globe. With the wave of omicron spreading across the Communist country, it's apparent that the CCP has started snorting from its own poisonous stash. Videos show apartment buildings being welded shut and quarantine tape plastered across the doors of families that have tested positive for the virus.[3]

American Authoritarianism Is Taking Root

Even with the predictable wave of viral Covid coming back around to the United States, very few entities here have advocated for a return to the masking and lockdown tactics. We are still a democracy despite it all, and perhaps the threat of the upcoming elections is mitigating any return to such strictures. Or perhaps there truly is a "cry wolf" moment at hand, and the entire canvas of pro-lockdown advocates have realized that the gig is up.

Yet from the start, the temptation to adopt Chinese-style authoritarian measures was too much for progressives and people of the Left to resist. The influence of China on American measures to stop the pandemic was patently obvious and very frightening.

Dr. Scott Atlas recounts a meeting with Anthony Fauci during his short stint on the White House Covid task force. Questioning the use of fear as a tactic, Atlas asked, "So you think people aren't frightened enough?" Dr. Fauci pushed back: "Yes, they need to be even more afraid."[4]

Petty Totalitarians Abound Unchecked

The citizen tattletales were everywhere. One Twitter user who claims to be a doctor declared: "An idea I've had is adding a reporting function to the covid tracer app. It would allow you to take pictures of rule breakers and send them quickly to MOH and you would be able to track the status of your report. I'm getting tired of having to write an email for every breach."[5] The eagerness of an entire set of people to willfully document and turn in their neighbors for the slightest infringements was something to behold.

A local Chicago CBS News reporter went to Twitter to scold and turn in a Jewish wedding: "The Hilton Chicago/Northbrook hosted a massive Orthodox Jewish Wedding tonight. 200–300 guests aprrox. No masks. No social distancing. During a pandemic. The state isn't allowing private banquet halls to be used/booked for weddings. How did this happen?"[6] Again and again, press conferences on every level of the government saw members of the media put on their best version of "turn in your neighbor." Rather than question government statistics and policies, media asked, Why aren't you doing more to close down businesses?

The Media Is Happy to Be in Bed with Authoritarians

By June 2021 Hollywood's assembly of propaganda was all set to roll out. In a choreographed number filmed for *The Late Late Show with James Corden,* pop star Ariana Grande joined the host in singing a tribute to Dr. Anthony Fauci. A flag of Fauci's face was unfurled by dancers, with a boom shot framing the city-street scene and then zooming in on the diva, who sang: "Once you've got the vaccine. Hug your family. Feeling so relieved. No lockdowns for me."[7]

The relentless push towards vaccination took a strident turn sometime towards the end of summer 2021. Massive legal initiatives were rolled out to prompt greater vaccine adoption. CDC Director Rochelle Walensky noted in October of 2021, "It is very important to get these people [the holdouts] vaccinated. There is a plan, should these people not want to be vaccinated, towards education and counseling."[8]

Information was withheld from the public again and again. Eerie FDA panels approving vaccines that were barely a year old gave the green light to administer vaccines to children without any significant vaccine studies. Said one member during the broadcast discussion, "We're never going to learn about how safe the vaccine is until we start giving it."[9]

California state authorities refused to give details on their tiers of acceptable levels of Covid for counties to reopen in January 2021. These health overlords in the Golden State just couldn't trust the public to understand quite yet. They said "they rely on a very complex set of measurements that would confuse and potentially mislead the public if they were made public."[10]

Dr. Leana Wen, who was featured almost daily on CNN providing Covid advice from a Team Apocalypse perspective, made it clear that vaccination wasn't really up for debate. Couching the "grandma killer" motif in softer language, she declared, "Being vaccinated is not just about individual choice."[11]

Building up to her infamous July 2021 First Amendment slap down, the White House press secretary Jen Psaki described what plans the Biden administration had in store to increase the number of vaccinated citizens. Shades of China for sure: "We will be going door-to-door to Americans who have not been vaccinated."[12]

While lockdowns in blue states and cities would become synonymous with authoritarian rule, the Canadian Great White North seemed to institute its own brand of Chinese-like overreach. One prominent member of Team Apocalypse in Toronto, Dr. Ellie Murray, rejoiced in government intervention throughout the pandemic:

> Trolls like to call me an authoritarian for my COVID takes, but I don't actually want the *government* to force *you* to protect yourselves. I want *us* to force the *government* to protect us all![13]

An October 2021 government edict declared, "Ottawa will prohibit all unvaccinated people from leaving Canada."[14] Canadian journalist Ezra Levant explained: "Even foreign citizens—if you're in Canada as a tourist, a student, a foreign worker, etc.—you literally won't be allowed to fly out from any airport."[15]

In Quebec, if you were unvaccinated, mandates required you do your shopping with a chaperone. An assigned "health warden" would usher you into any retail store. You could not be trusted to shop or make purchases unless you were under the watchful eye of government officials so they could escort you back to your dirty, unvaccinated abode.

The Trucker Rebellion Was Ruthlessly Crushed in the Great White North

Across Canada, truckers formed a massive wave of resistance to strict vaccination regulations. The threat was real: loss of job if they didn't submit. In early 2022, these truckers took to the streets in major cities across Canada, blocking roads and causing some disruptions to show their displeasure with these mandates. Canadian prime minister Justin Trudeau lambasted the protesters, implying they were putting lives in danger of Covid. He also labelled many of them racists. Canada's deputy prime minister, Chrystia Freeland, took it a step further in February: "If your truck is being used in these illegal blockades, your corporate accounts will be frozen, the insurance on your vehicle will be suspended."[16]

Back in the states, our health overlords continued to push for censorship. Not satisfied with his efforts to curb speech the year previous, Surgeon General Vivek Murthy took to Twitter in March 2022 to demand social media companies open their back end so they could start reprisals against American citizens:

> To create a healthier digital environment and safer future, tech companies must share what they know about #HealthMisinformation on their platforms. Only with this information can we work toward preventing harmful misinfo.[17]

Virtue-Signaling Businesses Kowtow to Government for Handouts and Profits

Corporations got into the game in solidarity with government mandates. Dunkin' Donuts promised free pastries to anyone who could show a vaccination card. McDonald's rolled out product branding on their french fry packaging promoting vaccines with colorful needles. One would hope someone at corporate headquarters would have seen the statistics noting that obesity was a key determinant in Covid outcomes. It's not a stretch to say that these two companies are more influential in Covid deaths than any mask-less face could ever be.

Intelligence Agencies Grab Citizen Data

More ominously, in Israel, where the omicron wave first appeared late in the fall of 2021, the country's intelligence agency was granted temporary permission to access the phone data of people in the country with confirmed cases of Covid.[18]

The rising hysteria and hyperbole continued into 2022. Dr. Morcease Beasley, superintendent of Clayton County Schools in Georgia, compared *not* wearing a mask to bringing a weapon to school: "We absolutely support the school district's decision to require masks of all even as we have rules for behavior including not bringing weapons. Why? Because of the safety of the whole community. Mask-wearing during a pandemic with a deadly transmissible virus is no different."[19]

These examples demonstrate that the authoritarian reaction to the outbreak that swept the world was a fatal export from China, arguably more harmful than the virus itself.

CHAPTER 32

What's Next

First, expect gaslighting. In February 2022, Impact Research, one of the top left-leaning strategy and polling firms in D.C., crafted a memo to Democrats about the current state of Covid politics. Right from the get-go this document will make you throw up in your mouth a little (or a lot).

"After two years that necessitated lockdowns, travel bans, school closures, mask mandates and nearly a million deaths..."

There was nothing axiomatic or necessary about any of this. This was a man-made disaster predominantly led by the elected and unelected officials of left-leaning blue states.

"It's time for Democrats to take credit for ending the COVID crisis..."

I'm not even sure how anyone can assert that with a straight face. We have fought Democrats (and many Republicans!) on these measures for almost two years now. It is pure gaslighting to claim that the Democrats had any semblance of power or will to "end" COVID-19. Many Democrats still do *not* want it to end. They strike a conciliatory tone next, but there's nothing altruistic about this memo. This is all about disastrous polling.

"Twice as many voters are now more concerned about COVID's effect on the economy (49%) than about someone in their family or someone they know becoming infected with the coronavirus (24%)."[1]

In other words, the more we talk about the threat of Covid and onerously restrict people's lives because of it, the more we turn them against us.

Well, at least they now admit that the restrictions were indeed onerous. There is plenty of gaslighting and bad math that follows in the rest of the memo, which will infuriate anyone on Team Reality. We can take some solace, however, in this point: they have inadvertently shown us the path to a return to normal—we have to mercilessly hold their feet to the fire!

Children Placed in Harm's Way Move Adults to Act

Public policy around child education appears to be a big influence. The failure of policies around our kids will be a prime motivator for our next mode of operations. We need to remind ourselves of how the "experts" were wrong time and again:

- Transmission of the disease—wrong
- Asymptomatic impact on transmission—wrong
- PCR testing—wrong
- Fatality rate—wrong
- Lockdowns—wrong
- School closures—wrong
- Quarantining healthy people—wrong
- Impact on youth—wrong
- Hospital overload—wrong

- Plexiglass barriers—wrong
- Social distancing—wrong
- Outdoor spread—wrong
- Masks—wrong
- Variant impact—wrong
- Vaccine efficacy—wrong

It Isn't Over until It's Over

April 18, 2022, may very well go down in history as the day that Covid died, or, rather, as the day the outrageous, never-ending, life-choking policies met a timely demise. A federal judge in Florida ruled on a case before her challenging the mask mandates handed down by the CDC. The ruling negated and voided that CDC order which was the basis for mandates across the country. Within hours, TSA, Alaska Airlines, United Airlines, and numerous other public transportation entities and companies dropped their mask mandate for employees and passengers.

It was a truly powerful moment. Videos online showed unmasked flight attendants coming down the aisle encouraging people to throw their masks away. Entire-plane selfies were taken mid-air as numerous pilots decided to end the mandate right there after it hit the wires. Twitter and other social media platforms burst alive with rejoicing (and some gnashing of teeth). Jeremy Faust, a prominent online physician with Team Apocalypse, lamented:

> The odd thing about my being disappointed in @united dropping its mask mandate is how many people who claim to love kids are totally cool with this meaning that a small number of babies will die of Covid, when we're weeks away from a vaccin[e] for all ages over 6 months.[2]

Always the same schtick—appeal to the general human inclination to *not* be called a murderer. For some of these folks, the end will never come. For others, it would take some time to adapt. One passenger tweeted out a very natural reaction to the dramatic change in policy: "I'm on a Southwest flight back to Sacramento and it was just announced by our pilot mask mandate is over. Flight attendant came through with a garbage bag to collect all of the masks. Feels weird!"[3]

It does feel weird. And that's an awful shame. The in-flight fights, reminders, admonitions, discomfort, nastiness, nervousness, and anxiety around masks were, it seemed, now behind us. The psychological damage was just being made known.

The mask mandate itself was set to expire within a few weeks, but the chances of its being renewed were ever-present on television Easter was just the day before the ruling, and newly installed White House Covid advisor Ashish Jha was making the rounds on the Sunday talk shows. "The pandemic is not over," he declared ad nauseam.[4]

A source contacted me just hours after the ruling and told me something was in the works. Shortly after the ruling, a TSA spokesperson declared that the TSA would no longer be enforcing the federal mask mandate on public transportation. Within minutes, full blog posts and emails were out the doors to customers of Alaska and United Airlines. The front page of the Alaska Airlines website's news page showed a flight attendant happily removing her mask: "Effective immediately, all Alaska Airlines and Horizon Air guests and employees have the option to wear a mask while traveling in the U.S. and at work. Masks are no longer required for travel and will be optional."[5] This was not just a quick turnaround—something had been planned.

My source informs me that the TSA and the airlines were waiting for this moment and had a strategy to get in front of any appeal that the DOJ or the White House might file. By the afternoon almost every major airline had announced they were dropping the mask requirement. More videos emerged of cheering on the planes, airline workers doing happy dances in the galley, and TSA employees grinning cheek to cheek.

"Nobody liked enforcing this. Nobody felt it was necessary or even doing anything," my source declared. "They just wanted it done with." Members of Team Apocalypse doubled down with outrage: Bob Wachter, the highly influential chair of the UC San Francisco Department of Medicine, tweeted: "Biden administration needs to fight this decision, even if [it] was gearing up to make the same call in a couple of weeks. Accepting a precedent that says that @CDCgov or other agencies don't have the authority to enact mandates during a public health emergency is enormously scary."[6]

The Media Wants Its Narrative Back

Ever-enmeshed in politics, reporters went looking for any death-laden message that might counter this lone judge's ruling. They attacked her age and origin (Trump appointee, clerkship for Justice Clarence Thomas) and lamented that this took away power from the federal government.

Jared Rabel on Twitter opined satirically: "I boarded a plane today with my son and mid flight, the pilot announces that the mask mandate is over. Flight attendants pulled off their masks and sneezed directly into their hands while screaming 'this is MAGA airspace.' My son turned to me in tears. I don't know what to do."[7]

The allusion to the recently finalized Jussie Smollet scam was a nice touch, but it didn't seem to seep into the thick head of *New York Times* reporter Victoria Kim, who messaged Rabel: "Hi Jared, I'm a New York Times journalist, I'd love to speak to you over the phone about what happened on your flight this evening. Can you please give me a call at [redacted] or let me know how I can reach you? Hope this isn't coming too late in your day. Thank you, look forward to hearing from you."[8] Rabel replied:

> Hello Victoria, I would love to discuss the incident at your earliest convenience. I was pretty upset about the whole thing. Unfortunately, it's satire that only someone at the NYT would believe. In my time of contemplation, I was wondering how your team deals with the multitude of false stories that you peddle out daily to use as political propaganda and if you could give me advice on how to take my satire to the next level? Best wishes.[9]

The *New York Times* had indeed been a front-runner among terrible publications touting exaggerated claims and front-page daunting visuals to spur more fear among the public. Rabel's reply reflects much of what Team Reality felt after the walls came falling down—we can't let this go down the memory hole, there must be justice served here.

By Tuesday, April 19, 2022, Uber had dropped its mask mandate. With one of the more stringent policies, super-woke Uber had readily used their 100 percent mask policy with force. Drivers could report passengers, and passengers could report Uber drivers for not wearing a mask. If a driver reported you for not wearing a mask, you would be asked to verify visually that you indeed did have a mask and knew how to wear one—otherwise your request for a ride was denied. Numerous passengers and drivers of rideshare apps were kicked off the platform for infringements of that policy.

The challenging thing is this: if the ruling is left to stand, then the CDC mandate and any mandate it "imposes" can be called into question in the future. The CDC had already suffered a massive and embarrassing defeat that went all the way to the Supreme Court. In 2020, the CDC declared that housing was a health threat and imposed a moratorium on evictions nationwide. This was found to be blatantly unconstitutional and a complete overreach. With its awful data, terrible (unconstitutional!) policies, and its ramrod ignorance of anything other than an apocalyptic narrative, no other government institution has suffered so much disgrace in so short a time.

Team Rationality Cannot Let Up the Pressure

We need to continue to pressure elected officials to open the floodgates on the response to the pandemic. We need hearings and publications to cover this with rigor. If we let it go blithely by without comment, we will face it again. We cannot let these unelected health bureaucrats near that type of power again.

We've explored some theories on why the plan to address Covid went off the rails. We surmised that certain forces have straight-up admitted to exploiting this vulnerable moment to fill a void and steer our ship of humanity in a very different direction.

As the pandemic (seemingly) draws to a close, I'm struck that it still feels that way. My guard is still very much up. Given all the fits and starts and restarts of government interventions, it still feels like there's an anvil hanging over our heads. That's indicative of the total loss of trust we feel towards our leaders who did little to stop the madness and less still in the way of an apology.

We're starting to regain some of the habits that were scorched away during the pandemic. I took my daughter with me grocery shopping the other day, something I avoided in the past two years because of mask stringencies. Social distancing and keeping a mask on my young children made shopping a joyless experience, so I did it without them.

I'm taking care to catalog the joys I experience in life now. I can't say I ever itemized those moments before, and now I fear that I may have forgotten something that was taken from us under Covid. There are days I fear we might not regain what we've lost.

Then again, I look at the amazing new life trajectories of people I've come to call friends from Team Reality. I've witnessed firsthand the bravery and courage needed to charge in when something is amiss. My wife Jenny and I had a child born to us during the pandemic, but we also experienced two miscarriages along with that birth. Still, we mustered on through all of the kid quarantines, forced masking, store shortages, school mayhem, and the deeply bitter members of Team Apocalypse calling for ever more of them.

It helps that in the end, we were proven right. The truth is coming out, and we feel vindication.

Now, it's time to fix a few things.

CONCLUSION

Someone broke America. Something wrecked the world. In this nightmare, neighbors have turned into agoraphobes, teachers fear their students, children are muzzled, citizens are censored, dystopian fictions have become reality, and unelected officials are creating a biometric police state. Oh—and people are masking up their cats and dogs.

Much of this insanity didn't *start* with the coronavirus pandemic. It was already latent in big government and most big corporations, and it won't end there. COVID-19 weakened the immune system of America revealing a decaying underbelly of confusion, panic, unease, and cowardice.

That cowardice turned viral as much as the virus did.

In fear, our health overlords (the unelected bureaucrats we turned over so much power to) threw away the pandemic response handbook. They said they were trying—beyond all reason—to protect every single person from the disease. They ended up protecting no one. From massive over-testing to universal plexiglass installs, to stay-at-home orders, to stay-away-from-school orders to mask mandates, to vaccine mandates, to some of the worst restrictions on civil liberties in American history, this is an epic story that poses big questions about America's future as a free society.

All of this happened with a virus that is considered moderate by pandemic standards. Covid is not a replay of the 1918 Spanish flu. It is not all that frightening by demographic standards. What is really frightening is how easily *they* were able to manipulate large numbers of *us* to wildly overreact and how uncertain it is whether we will ever get back our sanity. The panic went viral and broke the world.

It's still going on. In this book, I have sifted through the broken shards of the world around us, documented how we lost our ever-loving minds, and pointed out that *it's still happening*. I hope I've given those of us who remained sane the courage and ammunition to keep up the fight and make sure we don't get fooled again.

Team Apocalypse Admits It Wants to Remake the World

A global alliance of elite fixers straight-up admit that they intended to exploit the vulnerability of the pandemic moment to reshape the world. They enlist the help of like-minded health behemoths to jettison any hesitations of lowering the boom on all of humanity. This newly minted Team Apocalypse armed themselves with endgame threats of mortality to coax an already docile aging populace into obeisance. They bribed the masses to placate the obvious life-threatening impact of a jobless penniless family under their lockdown regimes. Corporations and elected officials fold easily in the face of alleged manslaughter and took solace in the knowledge that the free money scheme might actually imbue them with savior status.

The fearmongering was intentional. The ineptitude was palpable. The exploitation undeniable. The result? The fear of living life is part of us now—perhaps forever. Every human is labeled as a potential vector of disease. Anyone who diminishes the impact of Covid is a cold-hearted science denier. Anyone who questions the official "treatment" is committing murder.

The virus of the mind has done more to damage world than the COVID-19 could ever do. The panic Team Apocalypse sowed and nurtured went viral and broke the world.

To Get Back to Normal We Have to Get Back to Reality

Enter Team Reality. *Your* team. Our cause was getting back to normal. After one million deaths attributed to Covid we have to ask—did the massive measures really make a difference? The clear answer is that they did not. When all was said and done, the massive life-altering interventions made little difference in the outcomes.

Go back and look at who among your peers and family were on Team Apocalypse (those believing the end was near) versus Team Reality (those trying to shift us back into reason and rational thinking). As you catalog all of this, you should attempt to repair relationships strained by these tensions, but to do that you need to understand *why* they chose the team they did. I'm going to bet, with a few exceptions, you could have guessed which side they'd come down on for this.

My kindest interpretation is that many of the traits which compelled them to join in the fearmongering also make them empathetic and caring friends. Or perhaps they are cautious people by nature. I would say that a large portion of the people who joined up with worst-disease-ever crowd did so by default. After all, it is no easy thing to stick your neck out on a subject like this.

I recall waking early in the morning in March 2020 and thinking to myself: "What am I doing? What if I'm wrong? What if this really is as bad as they say it is?" That next morning Stanford professor Dr. John Ioannidis published an article to set the tone for the rest of the pandemic for me: "A Fiasco in the Making? As the Coronavirus Pandemic Takes Hold, We Are Making Decisions without Reliable Data."

He began the article on StatNews.com: "The current coronavirus disease, Covid-19, has been called a once-in-a-century pandemic. But it may also be a once-in-a-century evidence fiasco." He goes on to lament the lack of data on which we are making world-shaking decisions. He concludes, "If we decide to jump off the cliff, we need some data to inform us about the rationale of such an action and the chances of landing somewhere safe."[1]

Well, we jumped off the cliff and we fell hard.

I'm hoping you now have the tools to help friends and family back from the brink, bolster your own confidence in your own common-sense, and help you join the next phase of our work: making sure this madness ends. And that it never happens again.

ACKNOWLEDGMENTS

To my children, Kestra, McKaeln, Kaden, Hannah, Cordelia, Arya, Trinity, and Harley. You've endowed me with a lifetime of wonder and joy.

To my grandchildren, Malina and Alan. You are always on my mind.

To my brother Chris and sisters, Daria and Lauren, for your love and support.

To Aaron Ginn, who spurred me to always think bigger and waive off the haters.

To Don, who drove me to constantly find solutions and believe in myself.

To Jen Cabrera, for your immense patience and stellar editing skills.

To Kyle, for sharing your life-changing journey and inspiring so many.

To Scott Atlas, for your courage, trust, and eye for detail.

To Paul, for your strong encouragement and your love of family.

To Emily Burns, for your steady determination and vision.

For Gato, and your unrelenting spirit.

For Jay, for your kindness and fortitude.

For Amanda, and her courage to take up the pen with us.

For the many, many legions of friends and colleagues from Rational Ground and Team Reality: Len Cabrera, Clayton Cobb, Joshua Stevenson, Nathan, Megan Mansell, AJ Kay, Erich and Michelle Hartmann, Alex Rodriguez, Todd Lowdon, Karl Dierenbach, Len Cabrera, Daniel Horowitz, Shveta Raju, Woke Z, Scott Morefield, Ian Miller, Sam and Ellen Wald, Mark Changizi, Michael Betrus,

Nay, Lillith, ClownBasket, Emma Woodhouse, Phil Kerpen, Phil Holloway, Alan, Rusty Kuhl, Jeff Childers, Stinson, Rana, Matt Malkus, Jordan Schachtel, Jeffrey Tucker, Ben, Eric, Zach, Boutrous, The Robber Baron, Karina, Nick Foy, Megan Maureen, Jennifer Sey, Daniel Kotzin, Brumby, Ann Bauer, Jean Rees, Vanessa, Virál M., Julie Hamil, District AI, Kory Booher, Trish, Jenin Younes, Sarah Beth, Brian Kipp, Scott Morefield, and Tom.

Resources to Reclaim Our Ever-Loving Minds

This appendix includes multiple resources for readers to use, reuse, and share with others. We include multiple letters you might repurpose to send to a school board or summer camp, and even a letter to your lockdown mayor! We have also included multiple stories gathered from our sister website, CovidStoriesArchive.org, in appendix 2.

Letter to the School Board

Dear School Board,

Let's review.

Masks were optional from June of last year. It was left up to parent choice; even as school started in August and delta surged, you made the commitment to give parents a choice. Cases came down on their own, like we knew they would, because that's how viruses work. We knew cases would rise in the winter because we know the seasonality of viruses.

So imagine my surprise when after four months of no masks, we are back to mandating masks for just two weeks. I'm sorry, but I'm skeptical about the two weeks thing because the last time we were told to do something for two weeks is now nearing the seven-hundred-day mark.

And what was the basis for this? The Ohio Hospital Association wrote a note pleading with school districts to mandate masks because of hospital capacity. But did any of you ask them why they chose schools? Schools are one of the places that have the lowest rate of transmission. Did you ask them if they sent this to restaurants and bars? Arcades and bowling alleys? Hair salons? Did you ask them for data showing that masking kids would make a difference with hospital capacity? Did you question them about the extremely flawed mask study they used that has been retracted and debunked? Did you ask them if the type of mask matters since now we are being told cloth doesn't work? Did you ask them about the social and emotional downsides to masking? Or the way masks inhibit learning? Did you ask them if there are more children hospitalized for mental health reasons than COVID-19?

I could keep going. But if you didn't push back and just blindly accepted what they said, you didn't do your job. You didn't do the job that our tax money pays for. And guess what? My kids' job is to go to school and learn. My children's job is not to make sure there is enough hospital capacity. My child didn't fire unvaccinated healthcare workers. My child isn't responsible for the mismanagement of Ohio hospitals. Our kids did their part when they missed an entire fourth quarter of their school year. They did their part when they sat in front of a computer that you called school. They did their part when they were asked to give up sports and extracurriculars and to mask and to quarantine and to not have a graduation or a prom. Enough is enough. I refuse to have our children pay the price any longer.

And please don't insult me by saying, "No one likes masks, but if it keeps our kids in school…" Did you bother to ask why it keeps our kids in school? It's not because they work. We have two years of data from schools across the country and within our state that have been mask optional or mask mandated, and there has been statistically zero difference. Masks keep our kids in school because health departments told you that you won't have to quarantine if you wear masks. Students won't have to, and teachers won't have to. Masks keep our kids in school because you followed the rules. You are rewarded for following the rules that make no sense. Your compliance to a rule keeps schools open. Make no mistake—it is not the masks. The implication that masks actually keep anyone safer, especially kids that don't properly wear them, is strictly theater and a way to look like you are "doing something."

I would ask what the off-ramp is, but the problem with an off-ramp is there then can always be an on-ramp. If you set a metric, that metric can change at any time. Cases will rise at this time of year every year. We cannot mask and quarantine kids every year. Kids need normalcy.

My son was quarantined yesterday—I guess it was bound to happen at some point. But here's where I'm confused—yesterday was day five for him. He stayed at school until 1:00 p.m. Let's say he has it (he doesn't because he's already had it and has antibodies)—who are we protecting? He's been playing with friends all weekend. His sister (who he is with more than anyone) gets to stay at school. Who knows if she has it and is exposing her whole class? What about his dad who teaches? Hope he doesn't have it and is exposing all the teachers and students at Kidder. (My son tested negative today.)

Do you not see how ridiculous this all is? My child, who is struggling in math right now, had to miss time in school for no reason other than the guise of keeping people safe. And he's being punished for not wearing a mask. But funny enough, the person who has Covid was wearing a mask.

I know you are doing what the health department says, but at what point do you get to do your job? Push back. Demand an end date. Schools are not health departments. It seems that everyone can tell you how to do your job except for the taxpayers and the parents of the students. There are more things than Covid that kids need protection from.

Next time the Ohio Hospital Association wants you to do their bidding, ask them how many suicides and cases of self-harm have been reported since this all started. Ask them about usage of pediatric psychiatric beds.

It's time to give the kids back their life and education. They can't do this. Schools can't do this. And parents can't do this. And if it continues, I will find somewhere that's normal. Because it's out there. Maybe we should try it.

Signed,

Frustrated Moms of America

Letter to the Mayor of Boston

Dear Mayor Michelle Wu,

I believe that the descendants of immigrants are often the ones who can say with the most clarity what it means to be American.

I am the granddaughter and great-granddaughter of refugees. Following World War II, my maternal grandmother fled the ethnic cleansing of the Volksdeutsche in Croatia; in route to amnesty, she begged for bread from farmers who slammed the door in her face. My maternal grandfather, a budding intellectual and speaker of five languages, hid in the apple orchards of his village in Hungary, from where, after the communist regime declared an end to inter-village gatherings and banned him from attending school, he dodged Russian machine-guns and sought refuge in New York. Before arriving in Boston, my paternal great-grandparents managed to survive one of the most brutal genocides of the twentieth century. Now, all I have of their history is my surname, shortened to a more pronounceable combination of six letters, and, save for that ethnic "I-A-N" at its end, cleansed of any evidence of Armenian tragedy.

I think you and I agree that to be American and to be the [descendent] of immigrants means to understand just how much government matters. I think you and I also agree that to be American is to ensure that we are taking care of each other in the face of danger.

Thus far, other American cities have sacrificed their liberties in the name of government mandates that were supposed to be for the collective good. New York, San Diego, and Los Angeles have imposed some of the strictest lockdown measures since the spring of 2020. They continue to mask and distance children who, due to the exploitive hands of Big Tech, are already deprived of the tech-free connections that teach them basic empathy. They continue to place restrictions on the business owners who perhaps less than one generation ago escaped caste systems that kept them impoverished. They've continued to make second-class citizens out of the unvaccinated, with no success at stopping the spread of a virus that is more than 98% survivable for individuals without comorbidities. They've prioritized contact tracing over all other pressing responsibilities, like reducing crime, restoring trust with law enforcement, and re-evaluating economic policies that have skyrocketed housing prices and made their cities affordable to only the most privileged and elite of Americans.

All this, plus boosters—and these cities have not tempered COVID's relentless tantrum, with little to no reduction in case numbers, ICU hospitalizations, or levels of transmission.[1]

These policies are not only ineffective but wreak indefinite havoc on the livelihoods of those who they claim to protect. Repeating the same policies and expecting different results is commonly known as the definition of insanity. And I know that you, Mayor Wu, are not a woman of insanity.

I know that you, Mayor Wu, are a woman of innovation, that you are brave enough to learn from the mistakes of the aforementioned cities and disrupt their policies that attempt to control the uncontrollable. I know that you, Mayor Wu, are a leader who makes decisions not based on appeasing the interests of the establishment, but on preserving the liberties of the descendants of immigrants who came to America because they understood that sacrificing safety to live in freedom from oppression is far better than living in fear of an oppressor.

Sometimes, being American means sacrificing some of my liberties in the name of protecting my fellow countrymen; sometimes, being American is acknowledging where my individual freedoms end and where my civic duties begin. And if there were an outside force invading the city of Boston—one that aimed to exploit our fear, censor our lust for knowledge and intellect, enslave our grit, and assault our spirit—I would gladly lay down my liberties in the name of upholding the virtues of the land that granted refuge to my ancestors.

Such threats exist. And I know that you, Mayor Wu, can think of a far better solution than one that bans many Bostonians—the [descendants] of some of the most resilient, hopeful, and American peoples on the planet—the right to dine next to their fellow citizens, lest they relinquish their right to health freedom and inject themselves with a product developed by a multi-billion-dollar establishment that deceived doctors and knowingly enslaved millions of Americans to opioids.

I think you and I would also agree that we are a nation that so celebrates our accomplishments that the traumas of history often go unacknowledged; I learned of the 1956 Hungarian Revolution not from my textbooks but from my grandfather's first-person narratives; from my mother's mother, I learned to save the two-thirds-eaten remnants of a sandwich from my lunchbox; we covered Armenia for about a week in my junior year of history. From the unacknowledged traumas of my great-grandparents and grandparents, I know that to be the [descendant] of an immigrant is to experience in occasional doses what it means to feel unseen and unheard in our society.

I know that you, Mayor Wu, understand that so many are unseen and unheard in our society. And I know that you, Mayor Wu, have the power to see and to hear Americans like me, [descendants] who share our histories with our fellow Americans—too many of whom plug their ears, shield their eyes, and respond, with ill-informed idealism: "Don't be silly. Such oppression would *never* happen here."

Thank you for your time.

Sincerely,

Ms. Catherine J. Dorian

English Teacher, Writer, Entrepreneur, [Descendant], and resident of Greater Boston.[2]

Letter to My Summer Camp

Dear Camp Director,

We have read through your policies for this summer's camp session, and the answers to the questions in this letter will help us decide whether [camp name] will be a good fit for our children this year. It would be our oldest child's third summer and our younger child's second. They've very much been looking forward to a normal camp experience after many months of living in a city myopically focused on COVID-19.

We can appreciate that various competing interests and concerns have put you in a tough position. We also understand that your

Covid-related policies are the result of careful conversations and ever-shifting "guidance" from state and federal agencies. The changes in guidance this week alone have been head-spinning.

This year's policies appear to be more restrictive than they were last year, which is both puzzling and disappointing, given the following realities:

There is a range of effective treatments for those afflicted with COVID-19, and there are several effective vaccines for those over the age of eleven who choose to be vaccinated.

The virus poses a near-zero risk to children and teens in terms of severe outcomes.

The survival rate across age groups is 99.8 percent plus (higher among youth). Conservative estimates put total U.S. infections since February 2020 at over 115 million people; this number plus the 120 million people who have been vaccinated (with some overlap) contributes to a high level of immunity in the population.

COVID-19 is a seasonal virus that is not prevalent at Wisconsin's latitude during the summer months.

With this context, we object to several of the policies/measures you have adopted for this summer:

1) Requiring a Negative Covid Test for Camp Participation and (with High Schoolers) for Departure

This policy, which was not in place last year, makes little sense for a number of reasons.

First, many campers have likely already contracted and recovered from COVID-19, as our children did. We don't see the benefit or purpose in making children "prove" they aren't "positive" for a virus that they recovered from. It is highly unlikely that they will be reinfected, as there have been only seventy documented reinfections in the world. Your testing policy suggests that people are routinely reinfected after ninety days, which is not the case.

It seems your camp is adopting a "guilty until proven innocent"—or rather, "sick until proven healthy"—mindset. Children are being asked to make "not getting Covid" a daily goal, which is untenable, socially/psychologically harmful, and illogical. Redefining "sick" as "getting a positive test" and moralizing virus transmission is something we've come to expect of self-interested public health officials—not of you and your camp. If children are exhibiting symptoms of Covid-Like Illness (CLI) before camp, you should trust parents to respond accordingly. The quarantining agreement, while excessive, takes care of this. If a child becomes sick on the bus or at camp, we trust camp staff to respond accordingly, like we always have.

Testing of asymptomatic individuals is controversial even among prominent public health physicians. Testing a person against his/her will is unethical. Like all tests, PCR tests have a false positive rate. Moreover, PCR tests are very sensitive, and when the assays use a high cycle threshold (which most do), they are prone to detecting months-old, non-infectious virus. Under your policy false and "old virus" positives could keep campers from being able to attend. Testing high schoolers at camp and prior to departure feels more like a research study—or some kind of liability protection—than an actual concern for students' health and well-being.

Notably, other overnight camps are not requiring a Covid test for campers as a condition of participation [add names of camps here if you have examples].

2) Requiring Masking

Perhaps more puzzling than required testing is your requirement for masks on the bus and while walking into the dining hall, after campers have shown a negative Covid test. As demonstrated by data from around the world, including in the United States—and numerous studies—cloth does not stop viruses. There's no shortage of contradictory mask advice and claims, and even some of the most ardent champions of mask mandates are now calling for an end to such mandates, especially for children and teens. In addition, the World Health Organization has now admitted that the virus is airborne/aerosolized (and the CDC has also updated its site to state that infections can occur through inhalation at distances greater than six feet, which implicitly admits that it's airborne), which renders cloth masks even more useless.

We see that you're trying to create a "Covid-free bubble" with the testing, but we see no logic—or science—in forcing students to cover their faces on the bus or indoors. Even if cloth stopped viruses, the children will have tested negative, and adults have been given the chance to vaccinate. Further, last summer, our children's gaiters came home filthy. We don't want them wearing dirty cloths on their faces, nor do we want them spending time washing masks, especially when mask wearing is performative.

The truth is that schools across the country and in other countries have abandoned mandatory masking—or made masks optional in August 2020—without negative outcomes, including schools in Sweden and over one hundred public school districts in Texas. It may interest you to know that Christian Liberty Academy in Arlington Heights, Illinois, made masks optional last year. When we visited in March, almost no students were wearing masks, and only two staff were. The school had very few COVID-19 cases, even with that choice-based policy. This is not surprising and fits with data maintained by Dr. Emily Oster, professor of economics at Brown University, that shows required masking is associated with higher case numbers among staff and students in schools, regardless of community transmission rates.

Parents are the primary decision makers for their own children's well-being. Wearing masks should be an informed choice that belongs to the parents and their children.

Our daughter, in particular, experiences deep anxiety when asked or forced to cover her face. (In fact, she reported having a poor experience last year at camp with the limited masking.) Our son has bravely and successfully asserted his right to face freedom in stores and restaurants for months—which is an accomplishment in our mask-mandate county. The social and psychological messages that masks send are not harm- or value-free. Especially in a camp environment that emphasizes relationships between everyone involved, masks are a distraction and a barrier. The burden of superfluous masking is not one that campers should be forced to bear.

3) Privileging Vaccinated Campers

We were disappointed to read that your policies privilege campers who have been vaccinated for COVID-19. Even though our own kids have had the "typical" childhood vaccines, we don't recall your camp requiring vaccination records—or a flu or chicken pox vaccine—for camp participation. We don't oppose vaccination in general, but the push to vaccinate children for a virus that poses fewer risks to them than the flu is misguided. Privileging campers who choose a vaccine—and effectively punishing those who don't—is a highly questionable decision. It also strikes us as a form of coercion to say if campers get the vaccine, then they won't have to be subjected to testing (testing that no camper should have to undergo). Curiously, your policy says vaccinated high schoolers still need a negative Covid test to attend—due to potentially being asymptomatic—but don't need to test thereafter, while all other high school campers do.

We assume your camp's staff will have had a chance to be vaccinated. In that case, as three reputable doctors said in the *BMJ*, "The small risk posed to children by COVID-19 does not merit restrictions on any regular child activities in a context where adults are protected by vaccines."

4) Appealing to Virtue

Your email says that changes to the COVID-19 policies are "out of love and respect for others." Individuals have never been held responsible for ensuring that they don't unwittingly (that is, when they have no symptoms and have no reason to believe they are sick) transmit a virus to someone else, and love does not require surrendering one's own physical, mental, and emotional health to others' unreasonable fears or individual health needs. Campers and staff who are truly medically vulnerable to severe outcomes from SARS-CoV-2 infection should consult their own doctors and take appropriate steps.

In summary, we respectfully request that you reconsider both direct and indirect effects of the abovementioned policies on campers and change them to policies that are well supported by data and common sense. For each policy, state exactly why each measure is being undertaken, explain the underlying assumptions and values associated therewith, and cite relevant data and peer-reviewed research. There are any number of contractible/transmittable pathogens in camp environments, and campers participate in scores of activities that carry risk of injury or death. COVID-19 is on the very low end of the scale when it comes to severe negative outcomes for children. Asking parents and campers to pretend this virus is more dangerous than it is will cause unnecessary anxiety and may distract from potentially more dangerous threats.

Covid transmission, and the low risks associated therewith, have been moralized, sadly, and we have placed unfair, nonsensical burdens on children and teens throughout this pandemic. Please set them free from harmful, unnecessary protocols and useless mitigations so that they can have the normal camp experience they deserve.

Respectfully,

Stories from the Pandemic

One of the achievements we are proud of at Rational Ground is helping to fund, found, and launch a partner website called CovidStoriesArchive.org. Founded by Sam and Ellen Wald, the website helps capture and document numerous stories about people's experiences during the pandemic. With special permission we have reproduced some of these for you here:

"Stay Home, Stay Safe" Didn't Work for Me

My hometown locked down 3 days before my biopsy. 2 previous biopsies resulted in surgery for squamous skin cancer. I was told I'd have to wait 7+ months to get the biopsy & another line for surgery. I drove 5 hrs to a neighboring state, got biopsy & surgery within weeks. Then mask mandate occurred & I had to share a childhood trauma (hadn't even told my counselor) [because] it precludes me from wearing a mask. I fled to the city 5 hrs away, who had no mandate. My husband visited when he could. I lived in a hotel for 9 months until the condo we bought was available. My husband works in agriculture and can't move, I see him once a week. The work I was doing for 8 years: vacated. I'm lucky we had resources to find respite where I could live, but [it's] been a solitary existence for a year. I've tried to lead a productive life despite circumstances, but I'm changed.

Shelter Island

It's May 3rd 2020 and we'll be going into our 8th week of "quarantine" on Shelter Island. It's not quarantine in the real sense because none of us are currently sick. And I'm tired of people calling it that. Like a badge of honor. It's not.

I am scared and sad and angry. So so angry. This is no way to live. We can't just hide in our homes forever. Is that the plan? To just hide and let the days pass until either we pass or the "virus" goes away? Though as the days pass (slowly) the fear and the anger is lessening, but the sadness is becoming overwhelming. I'm sad that the future I thought we would have is a distant memory and what I see ahead is anything but rosy. I'm sad for my beautiful boy and all that he has already lost. I'm sad that I can't be my best self right now. The sadness is palpable and rises up through my body and gets stuck in my throat, like I want to cry and scream but I can't. Why can't I get through a day without feeling this knot in my stomach? How can I set a good example for my son? Why can't I get past this? I feel utterly hopeless.

Lockdowns and Mental Illness

March 13th, 2020 was almost a normal day, the last one I would have. I was sent home from my office that day where I worked with many people from all over the world daily in a testing center. That would be my last day of employment. Since that day, I have not left my home to go anywhere except outside or to the necessary doctor appointments. The media scared me to death with images of people dropping dead in the streets in China and Italy. Then came the news that obese and asthmatic people were some of the comorbidities resulting in death. That's all it took to turn my world upside down. I have not stepped foot inside a store, gas station, restaurant, or a family home since that day. My home has become my prison. I have suffered with health anxiety most of my life as well as PTSD from the Vegas shooting. Covid 19 was the final cherry on top of my mental illness sundae. Every night I dream of the mundane things I used to be able to do like walk through a grocery store or spend the day in my parents['] home. Such simple things that now feels other worldly. Then I wake up and the nightmare starts again. I have spent 2 birthdays alone in my home. I am now 30 and have no idea when I will ever be able to move on with my life, get married, or have children now. Every day I lose a little more hope. I'd give anything to have my boring life back even for a day.

Giving Birth in 2020 during COVID-19

I imagine I will always look back on 2020 as simultaneously the worst year of my life and the best. The best, because my son was born in May of 2020 and the worst because right as the world started to unravel, my father unexpectedly died from the cancer I thought he was successfully fighting. Nothing will ever break my heart more than the fact my Dad missed the chance to meet his grandchild by just a few months.

As we made our way in and out of the hospital each day to sit by my dying father's side in February of 2020, things were starting to get weird. We knew that a funeral was imminent, and we were hearing rumblings from Washington state about a virus killing nursing home residents and spreading elsewhere. We started to wonder if family and friends would make the trip to the funeral to say Goodbye?

The hospital started to limit visitors, but we had an "in." My Dad's wife was a nurse and an administrator at the hospital so we came and went without too much pushback. Knowing so many were denied this same opportunity to give comfort to their dying loved ones and were kept from overseeing the care their family members were receiving, will never not enrage me. Had I been put in that situation, I can almost guarantee I would have been arrested attempting to gain access to my dying father's bedside.

The timing of my father's death was such that we did have a funeral and guests did attend. We were lucky to be able to say our goodbyes with family and friends gathered in person. Just a few short weeks later, the majority of others would be deprived this important ceremony of closure for many, many months to come.

The weeks and months to my due date ticked by in excruciating slowness. Time had slowed down for everyone. My work had dried up, I was losing a lot of income. Spouses were no longer allowed to attend prenatal appointments or be present during sonograms. When I entered the hospital to see my Obstetrician I watched horrified as confused, elderly patients were denied the assistance of their care-takers (typically their adult children) for their appointments, forced to go inside alone and un-advocated for. Our temperatures were checked. We were handed a mask while being interrogated with a litany of health questions before being permitted access beyond the lobby of the hospital. I placed the mask in my purse.

During one of my final fetal testing appointments I couldn't help but overhear (she had the call with her husband on speaker phone) a woman in the next bed over lamenting being denied her husband's presence because she made the innocuous mistake of being brought in by her mother when her contractions started. Apparently the hospital would not allow you to swap out your support person. Whoever brought you in was who you were stuck with. He was floored at being denied the opportunity to witness the birth of his child and be present to support his wife in labor. When the nurses left I told her, "Discharge yourself, and then come back with your husband. Don't listen to them, they're not going to force you to stay or deny you coming back." She didn't seem to have any fight in her, so my suggestion probably didn't go anywhere.

Contractions started for me at 6am on May [date redacted for privacy], 2020. I waited at home for as long as possible before going to the hospital. The hospital had become a profoundly unwelcoming, totalitarian place that I wanted to avoid for as long as I could manage. I had done my research and was well aware what might happen if you tested positive for COVID-19 while in labor. I was also well aware of the high, false positive rate due to PCR tests being run at over a trillion-times more sensitive than was reasonable. (My work had all but dried up so I had a lot of time on my hands for research.)

We got to the hospital around 11am and my contractions were extremely painful. My thighs felt like they were on continuous fire. I was brought into a triage room but not yet admitted. They confirmed I was in active labor and were making arrangements for me to be admitted when I was told they needed to do a COVID-19 test. (Interestingly enough they did not ask to test my spouse or the doula I had hired to be there with us. Only my presence, the vulnerable, pregnant woman's presence was a threat to the staff.) I refused. They told me that if I did not take the test they would treat me as if I was positive. Which included not being permitted to have my spouse there. I did not agree to that and told them I needed pain management. I asked for gas and air (nitrous oxide mixed with oxygen) as I wanted to avoid an epidural if I could because epidurals can slow down labor which leads to increased risk of cesarean-sections, not because I'm a masochist. The nurses kept referencing printed pages with sections highlighted at every request I made, to check what I assume was the hospital's ever changing COVID-19 policies. I was told by one nurse they could not give me gas and air because COVID-19 was airborne.

I told her that she wouldn't deny an asthmatic an inhaler so why was she denying me an inhaled pain management drug. She said "it wasn't the same thing" but of course it was.

Hours went by and I still had not been admitted or given any pain management. I was left alone in the room and my pain continued to intensify to the point I couldn't take it anymore. After vomiting from the pain I sent my husband to get help and tell them I wanted the epidural.

They refused to give me an epidural unless I took the COVID-19 test. They withheld pain management as a means to coerce me into taking a medical test I did not consent to. I relented, desperate for pain relief. In active, excruciating labor, struggling to sit upright, they shoved a long swab so far up my nasal passage I could swear it was going to touch my brain. It felt like torture. I was told the test would take an hour to get a result back and that they were not allowed to re-enter my room for 30 minutes after administering the test. The reasoning for this "precaution," I can only assume is mass hysteria.

An hour came and went and no results, no epidural. I sent my husband back out with instructions to tell them to "stop dicking around and get me the fucking epidural." They had not previously told me they wouldn't give me an epidural until the test results were in, but they told us this now.

A new nurse came in, I guess the others had had enough of me. She took pity on me and gave me a shot of fentanyl which took the edge off and made my labor more manageable.

It was three hours before the test results came back. My results were negative. (As I had no fever and no signs of illness this was not a surprise, but it was a relief to have not been burdened with a false positive.)

The nurses withheld my admission for hours while I was in active labor, withheld the epidural I repeatedly cried out for, for hours, waiting for these results. To further punish me for not being a "compliant" patient they made me wait another whole hour for the epidural beyond this point as they put me through the admissions process that should have been completed hours prior. I finally got the pain relief I was desperate for (the fentanyl had long since worn off) after 6pm which was over twelve hours after my contractions had started and over seven hours since I had first arrived at the hospital.

I was lucky to get a delivery room at all with how long they made me wait to be admitted, I was told I got the last one. The nearby naval hospital's delivery ward had been shut-down for some reason related to COVID-19 and the hospital I was at had taken on all of their laboring patients. This doubled the size of their typical patient load, running the staff that was much too thin to handle it ragged. Despite this, to their credit the nurses did handle an emergency with my son that came around 11pm with great care and urgency.

My labor ended up lasting 28 hours, I didn't meet my son until late the next morning. The next day in the post-delivery room my postpartum nurse swooped in, demanding I wear a mask. Tired, angry, frustrated and in pain I snapped something to the effect of, "I will not wear a mask, I just had a baby, furthermore you forced me to take a COVID-19 test and it was negative so there is no reason for me to wear a mask. I will not!" She told me I only had to wear it while she was in the room, but I told her I would not and I did not. She of course was wearing her own mask. I must have startled her with the aggressiveness of my response, she didn't ask again.

Of course no visitors were allowed into the hospital, which frankly I was fine with. The last thing I wanted was the expectation of interacting with well-wishers, feeling as I did. I pressed to get discharged as quickly as I could. The idea of spending another night at the prison-like hospital was too much. We went home the next day.

Giving birth is stressful, scary and dangerous enough as it is. It is also supposed to be a joyous time. The response to COVID-19 has been so authoritarian, so myopic, so over the top, that it has robbed people of so much, including normal birthing experiences. It robbed each and everyone of us of missed experiences. The knee-jerk hysteria stole from us funerals, graduations, moments with newborn babies, and even just normality in a variety of situations including birth and face to face interactions. Where the virus itself has robbed many of their very lives, the response layered needless devastation on top of those losses with no benefit. Life is the collection of our experiences. We killed a year's worth of experiences trying in vain to stop a virus that was never going to be stopped by those restrictions. Worse still are the now-fatal cancer diagnoses that went missed in time for treatment, those that died from [being] too scared to go to the hospital to get treatment for their heart attacks, the delayed "elective procedures," the suicides and substance abuse fatalities spurred by lockdowns. These non-COVID19 deaths are laid plainly at the feet of humanity's desire to do SOMETHING even if that SOMETHING does nothing good.

What we're now left with now, over a year later, is a large swath of the population that are married to the idea of masks, lockdowns and fear of their fellow man so deep that it's going to take years for them disentangle themselves from these talismans and phobias. I can only hope the truth does come out and is so undeniable that those who need it most will have a reckoning of what they have done in the name of stopping COVID-19.

The Club DJ Who Lost It All

I am a club DJ from [state redacted here for privacy] that had the whole world in his hands. Good money, steady work [at] some of the best venues in the country, a beautiful (inside and outside) girlfriend that I always dreamed of having that I was getting ready to propose to, a family I still kept in touch with, and so many more amazing things. Life was beautiful. March 16th [state redacted] becomes lock-down and from there on out, my life changed forever.

I contracted covid19 shortly before lockdown and because I am obese, it did hit me hard to where I was bed rested for a couple of weeks. I have never been bed rested in my life nor did I ever feel like at 35 I thought I was going to die from a virus. I pulled through thankfully but the toll it took on me mentally and physically destroyed me.

I was absolutely paranoid the first few months of the pandemic especially [due] to a history of health anxiety. I wouldn't see friends or family, I wore a mask everywhere including gloves, washed my hands 100 times a day, sanitized everything constantly, and that paranoia is what ruined my life. Even when we were allowed to see others again, I wouldn't shake hands with anyone or go near anyone and being a DJ, that fear was killing me because I am a big people person.

Governor [redacted name of governor for privacy] became my public enemy number 1 with his lies and I let the hatred I have for him show more than any other emotion in my body during that time period.

Unfortunately the love of my life couldn't handle how I was being anymore and left me and that was the biggest hit I ever took in my life. That is something I will never recover from. I love her (even still to this day) more than I ever loved myself or anyone else and that will stay true for the rest of my life.

Because I am a DJ, money wasn't coming in and a very under-discussed subject through this pandemic was how low the amount of unemployment compensation was to workers of the nightlife industry. A "gig worker" would only get 231 [dollars] a week before taxes. 231 [dollars] is not even a quarter of what we in the industry would make a week. I began gambling my life savings online and at first, I was doing extremely well with it. Fast forward a few weeks later and it was all gone.

My family won't talk to me to this day for being so stupid and I don't blame them. The combination of losing the woman I thought I was going to marry and all the fear of covid, losing my savings, and fear that life would never be the same again, I began drinking heavily which I haven't done since I was in my early 20s and fell into a deeper depression than I could imagine. I attempted suicide on December 28th and was saved by one of my close friends.

Since then I have been doing my best to improve my life but it has been extremely difficult knowing that I destroyed myself and have nothing to show for it. Now that we are allowed to have regular nightlife and pretty much regular life again, I pray that I can build my life back to what it was before covid although the toll that it has taken on me. I'll never be the same again and I just sit here praying I can get my life back including the love of my life.

A College Experience during Covid

I was a little over halfway through my freshman year of college when Covid hit. I had worked my butt off during high school and was attending my dream school (a very prestigious and expensive university in the Los Angeles area), had joined a fraternity, made some incredible friends and was loving my life. School was hard, but I was learning so much and enjoyed my professors.

My parents own their own business and have dealings overseas, so they knew about Covid in November 2019. They actually sent me back to school after the Christmas break with a couple masks just in case. One of the guys living on my floor in the dorm was from the Wuhan area of China and our entire floor got sick shortly after classes resumed for the Spring semester. We were all young and healthy and shook it off within a few days. My parents were convinced that we all had Covid even though no one was talking about it here in the US at that time.

Then we received THE email. The one telling us that they were closing campus and we needed to be out of our dorms in two days. The next days were a blur as we all tried to finish our classes, pack up all of our earthly belongings and then make the trek back home. I settled into online classes for the remainder of the semester. It wasn't the same as in person class, but it seemed like the right thing to do as so little was known about Covid at the time. I was hopeful that I would be back in sunny California by summer.

Summer rolled around and campus was still closed. I decided to take a couple online classes as they were significantly less expensive than the normal tuition rate. I hung out with my old friends who were in the same boat and tried to stay positive even though I was growing restless. I was supposed to be enjoying a normal life as a college student and instead I was back at home.

The fall semester started and my university remained closed just like the rest of California. They decided to RAISE the already high tuition [and] charge us the Campus Life Fee even though you weren't aloud [sic] to step foot on campus. I decided to stay at home and go part time for the fall semester. The professors were trying their best, but I was surprised by how technologically illiterate they were especially considering the prestige of this university. I had heard stories from many of my friends that Zoom University at their school was a walk in the park. They would load up on 30+ credit hours and just coast through the classes because the professors didn't care and every test would be open note/open book. My university, on the other hand, limited the number of credit hours that you could take, limited the class sizes to 24 or less and seemed to increase the difficulty of the requirements and testing for the classes. I was miserable. I was still stuck at my parents house, taking ridiculously hard classes via Zoom with no end in sight.

My parents could see how miserable I was an[d] insisted that I go back out to California for the spring semester even if that meant I was doing Zoom classes from an overpriced SoCal apartment. At least I would be back with my friends. We found [an] apartment and I drove my car back just before Christmas. My parents were supposed to fly out and help me get furniture but my dad wound up catching Covid at his doctor's office (routine annual physical) the day after I left and so I had to rent a U-Haul and furnish my apartment on my own.

To my disappointment, my school remained closed for the spring semester so I settled into Zoom U from my apartment which I shared with 3 friends. It was hard spending so much time cooped up in my bedroom, but we were still able to go out and about in LA. There were many restrictions, and only certain things were open, but it felt like life might get back to normal soon.

By Easter, the four of us were going stir crazy and so we decided to go to Miami for a long weekend. We couldn't believe the contrast between Miami and LA. Everything was open, people were happy and life was normal. Back in LA, everyone was afraid and angry, people would shout at you if you dared to walk on the beach without a mask and things were still closed. My friends and I started talking about transferring to Miami.

I decided not to take any classes during the summer term and went home for an entire month. I was tired of being stuck in my apartment. I was tired of having to wear a mask everywhere I went, even outside. My roommates are my best friends, but we were on top of each other day and night and I needed a break.

In late July the university let us know that at long last campus would be open for the fall semester but that we would be required to be fully vaccinated. They said that limited exemptions would be granted. I have a preexisting medical condition and, as a result, I am not a candidate for the vaccine at this time. My doctor says that maybe I will be after some more information about the vaccine becomes available. My family wasn't worried about this because I am a healthy 20-year-old who has already had Covid and has some degree of natural immunity. I filled out the vaccine exemption paperwork and was both happy and surprised when my exemption was granted. I would be required to undergo weekly Covid testing (provided by the university) and to wear a mask at all times while on campus. I didn't care because school was open and things were looking up.

It didn't take long for my attitude to sour. The system set up to manage the weekly Covid testing didn't work. Despite dozens of attempts, I would be unable to schedule my test via the online system. When I decided to just walk into the testing center, I would be told that I couldn't be tested because I didn't have an appointment. After a heated discussion, they would reluctantly give me a test and my results would be emailed the next day (negative!). The following day, I would received a rather nasty email stating that I had failed to complied with the university's weekly Covid testing requirement and that if I were not tested within the next 24 hours I would be forcibly unenrolled from all of my classes and expelled from the school. I would call Student Health Services and they would locate my negative test and apologize for the confusion. This same scenario would be repeated on a near weekly basis.

Meanwhile it was becoming clear that things were far from normal on campus. Most of the restaurants on campus were closed. The microwave had been removed from the cafeteria because of "Covid" and they were only serving grab-and-go items like prepackaged sandwiches or tubs of cereal or Easy Mac. We were supposed to "cook" the Easy Mac by dousing it with a little boiling water.

If I was sitting alone in a private study room in the library and lowered my mask to take a drink from my water bottle, one of the librarians would run into the room, shrieking, "DO NOT LOWER YOUR MASK! YOU CANNOT LOWER YOUR MASK! NOT EVEN TO TAKE A DRINK!" If students objected and tried to point out that they were sitting alone in a closed room, they would be removed from the library by the campus security. I could list dozens of stories just like this.

Then the news broke that LA county was considering passing a vaccine mandate. I braced myself for the worst but was still hopeful that they would stop short of this draconian measure. Who was I kidding? It's LA and the mandate went into effect last month. I am no longer able to go out to eat, to Whole Foods or enter most stores. I have been completely blocked from living any kind of normal life in this city. The business owners are sympathetic to the fact that I have a medical exemption, but they are unable to break the rules lest they be fined. I now spend my days trapped in my apartment or in class and am counting down the days until winter break.

My professors are just loading me up with busywork. They frequently cancel class and it feels like they are just phoning it in. I recently told my parents that the only thing I have learned this semester is disappointment and how to be angry. When...people ask me where I go to school and I say the name, the automatic reply is, "Wow! That's a REALLY great school." I think to myself that they would be shocked if they actually knew what it's like on campus now and how far the educational standards have dropped.

I have decided to leave California. I have taken a leave of absence from my university and will be moving back home as soon as I am finished with finals. I am going to take a semester off and work for the family business. I am considering transferring to another school for next fall, but am honestly unsure if I will ever finish my degree. Covid has made a mockery of our university system and I am not sure if it will ever recover. My dreams of college and life in California have died a slow, painful death since Covid shut the world down back in March 2020. I am no longer angry. Life is too short and I am going to go start living it.

"My Trust of the Medical Community Is Gone"

It was exactly one year ago today that our family gathered on a conference call with the palliative team and our father. My brother and sister had been allowed to physically sit in the meeting with Dad, our first access to him since he'd been admitted 3½ weeks prior. It was deemed okay because he was leaving the next day for home hospice. To die.

Did I tell you he was blind? Yes. My father was blind.

The day Mom called for an ambulance he was checked into a local hospital in their tiny coastal town. He had kidney failure and pneumonia. They ordered him to be transported to a better equipped hospital four hours from his beloved wife and dog and home.

I was the only person who he felt comfortable sharing his sheer terror with through texts. "I'm f*cking terrified. Blind and alone to advocate for myself because it is Covid-times."

We called the hospital for updates multiple times a day. We played nice, said please and thank you, careful not to press further for fear they would take it out on dear Dad. Yes, we stayed inside the lines the medical community had drawn.

One year ago Dad flatlined during dialysis, so he made an exit plan. We heard him ask to come home over the line and all of us wept, but silently because strangers were in our sacred circle bearing witness as our hope bubble popped.

I will never forget. Never.

None of us should. My trust of the medical community is gone. They chose to follow the inane policies of government officials instead of the oaths they were sworn to protect and defend. I'm not sure how they come back from this. But maybe an apology is a good place to begin.

"A Caregiver to Young Adults with Developmental Disabilities"

I am a caregiver to young adults with developmental disabilities. I worked with a young person who lived with her mom. Mom is a retired nurse and at the beginning of the lockdowns was glued to the

TV for information. Her fear was reinforced in her child in order to make her understand how scary this was. Unfortunately, having the TV on most of the time with my "friend" hearing the constant fear-mongering left me trying to talk her out of believing that she was going to die from everything that the newscasters talked about. I was unable to do my job and was laid off in September. Some of my family members have unfriended me on social media for my "conspiracy theories" when I post scientific studies and truthful information that does not go along with their narrative of fear. I have chronic sinus issues affected by wearing a mask but was attacked twice for not wearing one and ended up using a shield in order to shop for groceries for my sis and self in peace. The anxiety that I feel when I am in public as a person who has worked and enjoyed being around others is one of the most difficult things I have had to deal with in my 6 decades on this planet. Knowing that my sis who has been housebound for 3 years due to health issues including chronic lung and blood clots is getting the shot floors me. I am afraid of the vaccine, not the virus.

Mask Mandates and Trauma

I need to share why mask mandates have been terrible for me. I have never shared this publicly, but I have to speak up because I know I'm not alone in my experience.

When I was 15 I was raped in the back of a pickup truck. The rapist covered my nose and mouth with one hand and held me down with another hand on my neck. At one point I jumped out of the truck and tried to escape, but he caught me. He caught me with his hand over my mouth and drug me back to the truck.

Every single time I put on a mask I feel creeping panic. It's been over 20 years since that attack, but the feel of anything over my mouth and nose instantly sends me back to that place. I feel bile in my throat and hands on my neck.

Mask mandates have driven me out of society. I avoid going anywhere that makes me wear them as much as I can. When my kids needed new shoes last spring and I had to take them into a store to try them on, I had a full panic attack in the shoe aisle and my husband had to pull my mask down and remind me I'm not there, I'm safe. This is what it has done to me, and I know there are other women like me out there.

A Positive Experience

I can't explain it. I have a lifetime history of chronic depression. In 2020 it went away, completely, and it hasn't returned. I live in South Pasadena, CA and life has never been better. I spend my days with my family, go on bucolic walks with my dog, I've gotten very good at my guitars, I got a Doctorate and a competitive scholarly award to go to India (which has been on hold). This is the opposite of suffering. I could do this forever if need be.

I Pray Daily Now

At first, the lockdown didn't seem like a big deal. I didn't have to travel for work which was a big relief. I was lucky enough to work from home and our company was doing well financially. As it went on, things began to deteriorate. First, my autistic son, who lived for going places like malls and other places, couldn't go anywhere, which built up his anxiety. Then my wife, who had a healthy skepticism of our public officials, became depressed because she was certain of impending conspiracy theories. Then my daughters saw their high school years trashed between lockdowns, masking, and remote learning. Their grades plummeted and they have lost their vibrancy. As time has gone on, I have seen a number of what once were conspiracy theories turn into reality. I pray daily for the health and safety of our family.

Waking from a Coma into a New World

In March of 2020 my father went to stay with a friend who had just lost his wife to cancer. The news was coming down that lockdowns were imminent to "slow the spread" and two weeks seemed like a good amount of time to stay with a grieving friend.

A few days later dad had a serious fall down a set of stairs into a cinder block wall. It was a severe TBI and the EMTs said it was one of the worst scenes they had encountered. They didn't expect him to make it to the hospital. They didn't expect him to survive surgery. He did both...but then he was in a hospital on lockdown. No one could visit. We couldn't talk with his doctors. He was in a coma for a month and during that time my stepmother camped out at a nearby hotel hoping that some day she could just see him. Just know he was alive.

We worried every day. Will he survive the coma only to be killed by covid? We tried our best to get updates from the busy nurses. He woke from the coma but was too weak to hold a phone. My stepmom viewed him from a window. And waved.

For over a month we worried and felt like life was standing still. No help, no support, no words of encouragement. It was a new world and no on[e] seemed to know how to move ahead. Time stood still truly for all of us. And when my dad woke up he could not comprehend how much had changed in just one month...he woke up to a literal new world. Like something out of a sci fi novel and he could not comprehend why the world now was so scared of dying that no one was living.

The Burdens on a Young Girl

I'm the mom of a 5 year old girl. She was 4 when the pandemic started. I watched my child, who strangers often commented was the happiest child they had every seen, become sad, withdrawn and irritable due to covid lockdowns. After not leaving the house for two months she was a different child. We were extremely fortunate to have neighbors across the street with similarly aged kids that my daughter got to play with. I honestly believe it was their friendship and relationship that saved my daughter.

My daughter was able to go back to daycare, but in a mask and "socially distanced" from her friends. It's better [than] nothing but definitely not great. Now that adults have been vaccinated she'll be going to school in a mask that the adults around her aren't forced to wear.

The way we have treated kids throughout this pandemic has been an abomination. I'm sure many people will forget but I never will. I will never again believe that public health experts are trustworthy.

Personally, I feel politically lost. Previously I considered myself a democrat but after seeing how they have treated minorities and children I don't think I can ever say that again. I have no trust in the government. I've always been skeptical [but] the pandemic has taken that to an entirely new level.

"People Are Literally Dying to Avoid Contracting the Coronavirus"

Posted at Rational Ground by our colleague Michael Simonson.

"Let's go to the hospital," Dalia Ayala told her fiancé, and my friend, Noe Borjas, after he complained to her in mid April of pain on the left side of his body.

A month earlier, while struggling with a liver-related health issue, Borjas reluctantly allowed Ayala to take him to the emergency room near their Northern New Jersey apartment, just across the Hudson River from Manhattan. Since his discharge in mid-March, the coronavirus had rapidly spread across the New York City tri-state area, killing over 9,000 people.

Now, Borjas refused Ayala's request to go to the hospital. "I'm afraid they are gonna leave me there by myself. You won't see me,"

Ayala remembers him saying. "I'm afraid of this (Covid) stuff going around."

Four days later, on April 15, Borjas's condition deteriorated to the point that Ayala had no choice but to call an ambulance to take him to the emergency room. Due to Covid-related regulations, Ayala had to stay home.

Borjas' doctors called Ayala early the next morning. "They were waiting for the surgeon to come because he had internal bleeding," Ayala recounts. "One of his vessels ruptured and that was causing the problem" (the doctors told Ayala that Borjas' hospitalization was unrelated to Covid).

Ayala called the hospital back a few hours later. She was connected to a nurse named Bethany. "Can you tell him that Dalia loves him?" Ayala asked.

Bethany called Ayala back the same day. "(She) let me know that he was gone," Ayala says. "When she told me what happened, I asked her, 'Did you tell him what I ask?' She said, 'Yes, that's when he relaxed.'"

Borjas was dead. He was 48.

"If your body is not right," Ayala advises now, "listen to that and go to the hospital, even if you're afraid of going."

The New York Times reported on December 13 that there have been at least 356,000 more deaths in the United States than usual since the start of the coronavirus pandemic.

While the majority of this year's excess deaths were from Covid-19, more than a quarter were related to other causes, including diabetes, Alzheimer's disease, high blood pressure and pneumonia, *The Times* noted.

Many of those non-Covid excess deaths, reporter Denise Lu wrote, are most likely indirectly related to the virus and caused by disruptions from the pandemic.

Lu identified three such disruptions, including strains on health care systems and inadequate access to supplies like ventilators.

The third deadly disruption identified by Lu may have cost Noe Boras his life: People avoiding hospitals for fear of exposure to the coronavirus.

The fatal trend emerged soon after the start of the pandemic. In early April, *ProPublica* reported that at-home death rates had spiked in New York City; parts of Massachusetts, Michigan, and Washington State; and other regions.

While some of those spikes may have been from people infected with Covid-19 who didn't seek treatment or were instructed to shelter in place, *ProPublica* observed, "It's possible that the increase in at-home deaths reflects people dying from other ailments like heart attacks because they couldn't get to a hospital or refused to go, fearful they'd contract COVID-19."

That same month, the medical publication *STAT* provided additional evidence that the at-home death spike was due, in no small part, to a lack of treatment for non-Covid conditions.

Cardiologists across the U.S., *STAT* reported, had become "worried about a second wave of deaths caused indirectly by Covid-19: patients so afraid to enter hospitals that they are dying at home or waiting so long to seek care that they're going to suffer massive damage to their hearts or brains. Some call it 'a virus of fear.'"

STAT referred to an early April survey of nine major hospitals that showed the number of severe heart attacks being treated in U.S. hospitals had dropped by nearly 40% since the coronavirus began spreading widely in March.

"The whole community is discussing this, asking where are all of our patients?" Martha Gulati, the chief of cardiology at the University of Arizona, told *STAT*. "There's nothing we've done overnight that has cured heart disease."

Gulati added that patients were coming in so late that they had massively damaged hearts, including heart muscles that have ruptured. "That was something I'd only seen before in textbooks, to study for exam questions," she said. "Now we're seeing those cases because people are putting off care."

Mitchell S.V. Elkind, an attending neurologist at NewYork-Presbyterian, a New York City hospital at the epicenter of the pandemic, revealed to STAT that about half as many patients as normal were in his stroke unit. "People with stroke symptoms really need to know they should come in for treatment" immediately to limit brain damage and the risk of permanent paralysis, he said.

Boykem Bozkurt, the president of the Heart Failure Society of America and professor of medicine at Baylor College of Medicine, echoed Elkind's concern to STAT. "If anything, we would expect higher rates," he said. "We are not seeing the number of patients we should be seeing."

Many of the "missing" patients from American hospitals "may indeed be dead," reporter Usha Lee McFarling theorized, pointing to a report by New York City's EMTs. Between March 30 and April 5, the EMTs fielded 1,429 cardiac arrest house calls in which patients could not be revived, an eight-fold increase from the same period a year earlier.

"While some of the fatalities were likely caused by the novel coronavirus," McFarling wrote, "others may have been caused by untreated cardiovascular disease or stroke."

Bozkurt agreed. "I think globally, we are going to see adverse trends in...cardiovascular deaths due to our patients not seeking care because of Covid," he speculated.

A New York Times report from May offered additional examples of people delaying potentially life saving treatment to avoid contracting Covid.

For "time-sensitive procedures like cardiac catheterizations, cancer surgery and blood tests or CT scans to monitor serious chronic conditions," reporter Katie Hafner wrote, "doctors now find themselves spending hours on the phone trying to coax terrified patients to come in."

Hafner cited a review by the insurance company Cigna Corporation of its claim and pre-authorization data for seven acute conditions, including heart attacks, appendicitis and aortic aneurysms. The review found declines ranging from 11 percent for acute coronary syndromes to 35 percent for atrial fibrillation in the rate of hospitalizations over a recent two-month period.

"People are saying: 'So I'm having a heart attack. I'm going to stay home. I'm not going to die in that hospital,'" Dr. Marlene Millen, a primary care physician at the University of California, San Diego, told Hafner. "I've actually heard that a few times."

Like *STAT*'s McFarling, Hafner referenced EMT data showing a link between the drop in non-Covid care and the rise in at-home deaths. In Newark, New Jersey, Hafner reported, emergency medical services teams made 239 on-scene death pronouncements in April, a fourfold increase from April 2019.

Fewer than half of those additional deaths could be attributed directly to Covid-19, according to the president and chief executive of Newark's University Hospital.

In some parts of the country, the increase in at-home deaths continued into the summer.

Between March and August, *The Charlotte Observer* reported, the number of people found dead in their homes in North Carolina's Mecklenburg and Orange counties rose 35% and 31%, respectively.

In Orange County, none of the deaths were linked to Covid-19.

"Fear (of contracting COVID-19) absolutely played a major role in (the increase in at-home deaths)," Joey Grover, the county's medical director for emergency services, told *The Observer*. "Just because COVID is happening doesn't mean baseline heart disease has gone away. I think there are fewer people seeking care."

A sizable portion of Houston and Los Angeles' summer at-home deaths were also caused by people delaying treatment for non-Covid conditions, according to reports by *ProPublica* and *The Los Angeles Times*, respectively (though you have to scroll way down both articles—and literally to the bottom of the *LA Times* story—to read about it).

"Normally these patients would have called us earlier on, and now they are waiting too long because maybe they don't want to be transported to a hospital," Houston Fire Department Senior Capt. Isabel Sky-Eagle told *ProPublica*. "Now we're catching them when they're already in cardiac arrest, and it's too late."

In one South Carolina county, the elevated at-home death rate lasted into the fall.

"Call volume to the (Anderson County) county coroner's office has been 'through the roof' (for at-home deaths) since the pandemic began," according to an October report by local news station *WYFF*.

"The coroner's office links the increase in at home deaths," Devlin added, "to people in need of medical care electing not to visit the hospital due to fears of contracting COVID-19."[1]

Immunocompromised

Above we've discussed at length the reasons why people go along with the flow of things. Why did so many of our fellow citizens don the mask or take the shot without asking a single question? Why didn't we take our masks off when it was determined that what we did for two years amounted to "facial decorations"? One interpretation might be kindness and sensitivity. Nobody likes confrontation, and many people are perfectly willing to make sacrifices to meet some personal feeling of "helping." So it was that when the masks came off and the vaccine waned, we were left wondering aloud: What about those who have need to fear the disease? Amongst us are those with seriously immunocompromised bodies. What obligation do we have to these folks to continue with the mitigation if mitigation helps stem their disease and fear? Our colleague Alex Lieske wrote a piece for us at RationalGround.com that we reproduce in whole for your elucidation:

"I'm Immunocompromised, and I've Never Asked Others to Protect Me"

"Get that child to the hospital RIGHT NOW."

Those were the words that rang in my mother's ears when she picked up the phone at midnight in the winter of 1984. She all but threw my father out of bed as they hastily got dressed, told my older brother to hold down the fort (he was 13), scooped me up (I was 5 years old at the time), and carried me to the car. I'd had a fever of 102 or above for 3 straight days. What seemed like an ordinary seasonal bout of the flu turned out to be a fight for my life. I was yellow (jaundiced) and anemic, and my spleen was considerably enlarged. All I remember is how calm my parents were while getting me to the hospital and their smiles and promises of all the ice cream that I could eat as we were met at the emergency room door. The hospital staff, learning about my bloodwork, thought that a dead kid was being delivered into their arms.

I have hereditary spherocytosis. It's a blood disorder that causes my red blood cells to be shaped like spheres instead of flattened discs. The spleen normally helps to filter bacteria and damaged cells out of the blood stream, but the strange shape of my red blood cells sends the spleen into overdrive. I truly can't remember the specifics of my bloodwork, but it was bad. Very bad. Luckily, I was out of the hospital in a few days but went back in with a similar event when I was 7 years old. At 8 years old, I finally had my spleen removed. As I had entered elementary school and had begun playing contact sports, my enlarged spleen had become more dangerous, as it could more easily burst (I actually had two spleens, which I believe makes me a medical marvel, but they both had to go).

I am one of an estimated 10 million people in the United States with a compromised immune system. I don't feel any different than anyone else, and it doesn't hold me back. I went on to play Division I lacrosse at Duke University, and I'm now married with three young children. But it's something that I know elevates my risk in certain scenarios, and I'm wary of it. Every day, from the time I had my spleen removed at 8 years old until I graduated from college, I took amoxicillin to help bolster my immune system and fend off infections. I've gotten every vaccine known to mankind. To limit my risk, I continue to work out by boxing or running 4–5 days per week, and I try to eat healthy (outside of my childish, guilty pleasure of Chips Ahoy cookies and milk…nearly every night). Understanding my individual risk, I take measures in my daily life to make sure I'm as healthy as possible to help boost my immune system. This is my individual risk, and my individual risk alone; no one, and I repeat, NO ONE is responsible for my health other than me. And on the flip side, others are responsible for their own health. This is how I've always lived my life.

Then 2020 hit, and along came COVID-19. At first, the response was unified as we learned more about this infectious, aerosolized virus that no human intervention measures can stop (AIER lists over 30 studies showing the ineffectiveness of lockdowns, for example). As time went on, it seemed that the response was becoming more about politics and "winning" than about the virus. Every psychological trick in the book has been tried, some to great success ("my mask protects you; your mask protects me," "stay home, save lives," it's all for "the common good"). Despite my issues with almost all of the fear messaging over the past year, the one that really made my blood boil was the mass vaccination campaign that broadly weaponized the "immunocompromised" as a reason that everyone, young and old, needs to be vaccinated, with an emergency use vaccine (until very recently, and 2 of the 3 vaccines are still under emergency use authorization), against this terrible disease.

Universities started to require vaccination to return to on-campus learning, and businesses are coercing employees, as well. In one of the more divisive speeches I have ever heard, President Biden used his bully pulpit to shame and ridicule the unvaccinated, erroneously calling them a danger to the vaccinated. Then came the emails from my kids' schools, one stating that they are still determining whether or not to require the vaccination this school year. Another implied that the only way to return to normalcy is through 100% vaccination of the student body. My children are 10, 9, and 6, so this sent chills down my spine. My answer, put bluntly, was "absolutely not."

As I said before, I am pro-vaccine. I'm also pro-individual liberty. And, most of all, I'm pro-critical thinking. Why on earth are we coercing and pressuring parents into vaccinating kids and adolescents with an EUA vaccine (the full approval for Pfizer is only for 16+)? Remember when we did everything out of "an abundance of caution"? Does the precautionary principle not apply here? Are these schools feeling political pressure, or are they so far down the fear-narrative rabbit hole that they don't realize that COVID-19, thankfully, isn't dangerous to children?

As world-renowned epidemiologist and physician-scientist John Ioannidis said, and Scott Atlas echoed, the risk to children is "almost zero." Most school-aged kids across Europe have been going to school normally, without masks or distancing, for the past year without issue. In Sweden, at the height of the pandemic hysteria in March 2020, 1.95 million kids younger than 16 attended school without masks or distancing through June. The result? 15 developed severe COVID-19 and none died…out of 1.95 MILLION. This happened almost everywhere in Europe for children; how irrationally fearful have we become in the U.S. that we are not able to think critically about this when it applies to schools and vaccines for young kids?

It's possible to be pro-vaccine while also wanting to see more long-term results in regards to the usage of COVID-19 vaccines in children. As stated in an opinion piece written by Vinay Prasad, Wesley Pegden, and Stefan Baral: *"Unlike for adults, the rarity of severe covid-19 outcomes for children means that trials cannot demonstrate that the balance of the benefits of vaccination against the potential adverse effects are favorable to the children themselves. In short, given the rarity of severe clinical courses and limited clarity of risks, the criteria for emergency use authorization do not appear to be met for children."*

The vaccine appears to be effective in limiting severe cases and hospitalizations, so if you are vaccinated, you should have no concerns. And if you're a parent, the exceptionally low risk profile of the 0–17 age demographic should put you at ease as well. But at the end of the day, this should be about the choice of the family and the child and their personal pediatricians; any type of pressure or coercion is unacceptable and continues to erode our trust in public health, which is already going to take a generation to repair.

As an immunocompromised individual, I NEVER asked for this, and there are millions like me. It's not the government's job to protect my health; it's the government's job to protect my freedom, liberties, and rights. How dare we keep children out of school for a year (or more) using people like me as the reason, without our consent? How dare we mask and distance our children and close schools when globally—and domestically—we have data showing it's completely unnecessary (in fact, mask-optional schools showed lower transmission)? How dare we use children as shields for adults? If it's not clear, this has never been about students or their health, but it has everything to do with institutions trying to appease the mob and avoid any conflict. That's no longer acceptable, if it ever was. Kids are not responsible for the irrational fears of adults. Children unequivocally aren't responsible for my health, and I never would ask them to be.

Adults, we have failed children for over a year. And now, holding kids' educations ransom until they get an EUA vaccine, when they are at lower risk from COVID-19 than influenza, is the one of the worst things humanity has done, and these measures, without a doubt, disproportionately affect the disadvantaged and marginalized. And don't get me started on the teachers' unions.

We can start to repair the damage we've done before it's too late. The school year just started, and already we are seeing disruption and quarantines in the name of "safety." There are universities, including my alma mater, Duke University, going fully-remote, with mask mandates indoors and out, despite 95%+ vaccination rates on campus. What is the off-ramp? And if we are trying to increase uptake of vaccinations, I can assure you that this is the exact opposite strategy that should be employed.

It is time to reshape the narrative, add context to the COVID-19 risk profile that has been hidden for a year, and start to promote self-responsibility and accountability when it comes to one's health. And, one more time for those in the back, you are not responsible for my health or my family's health, and I am not responsible for yours. Let's start acting like civil adults again. It's time for humanity to move forward for the sake of our most valuable asset, our children.[2]

Introduction: Debunking the Myths of Covid

1. Omnipotent Moral Busybody (@OBusybody), "Masking children to reduce the spread...," Twitter, May 7, 2021, 11:07 a.m., https://twitter.com/obusybody/status/1390714874897084416?lang=en; Jack Davis, "Facebook Suspends User for Doubting the Practicality of Masks on Children, Now Social Media Platform Is Facing a Monster Suit," The Western Journal, July 18, 2021, https://www.westernjournal.com/facebook-suspends-user-doubting-practicality-masks-children-now-social-media-platform-facing-monster-suit/.

   Here's the complete list:

   Children are at very low risk from COVID-19.

   Children spread COVID-19 much less than adults.

   Asymptomatic children rarely spread COVID-19.

   Teachers do not face an increased risk from children.

   Schools have not driven the spread of COVID-19.

   The effectiveness of masks is not conclusive.

   Masking children correctly is unrealistic.

   Improper masking is common and unsanitary.

   Many places do not require masks on children.

   Schools without masks have not fared worse.

   Masks can hinder speech development in children.

   Deaf and disables children struggle to learn with masks.

   Masking can often cause headaches and fatigue.

   Some masks contain toxic chemicals.

   Masking can cause a variety of other health issues.

2. "Press Briefing by Press Secretary Jen Psaki and Surgeon General Dr. Vivek H. Murthy, July 15, 2021," The White House, July 15, 2021,

https://www.whitehouse.gov/briefing-room/press-briefings/2021/07/15/
press-briefing-by-press-secretary-jen-psaki-and-surgeon-general-dr-viv
ek-h-murthy-july-15-2021/. Psaki gave a glimpse of how the scheme
works: "We are in regular touch with these social media platforms, and
those engagements typically happen through members of our senior staff,
but also members of our COVID-19 team." The next day she revealed
that the far-reaching effort targeted multiple posts on multiple social-
media sites: "You shouldn't be banned from one platform and not
others." "Press Briefings by Press Secretary Jen Psaki, July 16, 2021,"
The White House, July 16, 2021, https://www.whitehouse.gov/briefing
-room/press-briefings/2021/07/16/press-briefing-by-press-secretary-jen
-psaki-july-16-2021/.

Psaki, along with Biden's surgeon general Vivek Murthy, insisted that
social-medical platforms "measure and publicly share the impact of
misinformation on their platform." In addition, Biden and Murthy
directed companies to "create a robust enforcement strategy that bridges
their properties and provides transparency about the rules." The White
House published an entire 22-page advisory with instructions on how
social media companies should remove posts with which Murthy and
Biden disagree. "Press Briefing by Press Secretary Jen Psaki and Surgeon
General Dr. Vivek H. Murthy."

Chapter 1: Interventions Have No Costs! WRONG.

1. Paul Simon, "Dr. Fauci—Asymptomatic NOT Driver of Epidemics,"
   YouTube, October 11, 2020, https://www.youtube.com/watch?v=JIOz
   No3ZWXY.

2. Kajanan Selvaranjan et al., "Environmental Challenges Induced by
   Extensive Use of Face Masks during COVID-19: A Review and Potential
   Solutions," *Environmental Challenges* 3, no. 100039 (April 3, 2021),
   https://www.ncbi.nlm.nih.gov/pmc/articles/PMC7873601/; see also
   Yiming Peng et al., "Plastic Waste Release Caused by COVID-19 and
   Its Fate in the Global Ocean," *Proceedings of the National Academy of*

Sciences of the United States of America 118, no. 47 (November 8, 2021), https://www.pnas.org/doi/10.1073/pnas.2111530118.

3. Jean Benjamin, "Disposable Face Masks, an Ecological Disaster in the Making," Medium, November 10, 2020, https://medium.com/@jeanb enjamin/disposable-face-masks-an-ecological-disaster-in-the-making-40 e698512afb.

4. "The Potential Impact of the COVID-19 Response on Tuberculosis in High-Burden Countries: A Modelling Analysis," Stop TB Partnership, May 2020, https://stoptb.org/assets/documents/news/Modeling%20Re port_1%20May%202020_FINAL.pdf.

5. M. Harvey Brenner, "Unemployment, Bankruptcies, and Deaths from Multiple Causes in the COVID-19 Recession Compared with the 2000–2018 Great Recession Impact," *American Journal of Public Health* 111, no. 11 (November 1, 2021): 1950–59, https://ajph.aphapublications.org /doi/full/10.2105/AJPH.2021.306490.

6. "President Donald J. Trump Is Providing Economic Relief to American Workers, Families, and Businesses Impacted by the Coronavirus," The White House, March 27, 2020, https://trumpwhitehouse.archives.gov /briefings-statements/president-donald-j-trump-providing-economic-rel ief-american-workers-families-businesses-impacted-coronavirus/.

7. Cole Little, "WATCH: Joe West Snitches on Nationals GM for Not Wearing Mask, Has Him Kicked Out," Cubs HQ, September 6, 2020, https://www.cubshq.com/cubs-baseball/update/watch-joe-west-snitches -on-nationals-gm-for-not-wearing-mask-has-him-kicked-out-28767.

8. Matt Snyder, "Dodgers Star Justin Turner Pulled from World Series Game Due to Positive COVID Test," CBS News, October 28, 2020, https://www.cbsnews.com/news/justin-turner-covid-dodgers-world-ser ies/.

9. Associated Press, "NFL Could Become Trendsetter for COVID-19 Policies: Fewer Tests for Vaccinated," Newsmax, December 21, 2021, https://www.newsmax.com/finance/streettalk/virus-outbreak-nfl-futu re/2021/12/21/id/1049468/.

10. "Covid-19: PM Says 'Now Is the Time to Take Action,'" BBC News, October 31, 2020, https://www.bbc.com/news/av/uk-54761534.

11. Reuters, "Google, Apple Unveil Built-In COVID-19 Exposure Notifications," *New York Post*, September 1, 2020, https://nypost.com /2020/09/01/google-apple-unveil-built-in-covid-19-exposure-notificati ons/.

12. Here's the result of contact tracing for San Diego county between June 2020 and May 2021. The percentage denotes the share of cases at the location.

> Bars and Restaurants—7.3%
>
> Casinos—0.8%
>
> Group Gatherings—2.4%
>
> Gyms—0.5%
>
> Hair Salons or Barbers—1.8%
>
> Places of Worship—2.0%
>
> Protests—0.0%
>
> Retail locations—9.5%
>
> Workplaces—31.6%
>
> Schools—4.6%
>
> Household Exposures—36.1%
>
> Air Travel-related Exposures—13.7%.

This list is from "COVID-19 WATCH: Weekly Coronavirus Disease 2019 (COVID-19) Surveillance Report," San Diego County, June 22, 2021, https://web.archive.org/web/20210626174335/https://www. sandiegocounty.gov/content/dam/sdc/hhsa/programs/phs/Epidemiology/ COVID-19%20Watch.pdf.

This seems like some very useful data. There's one hitch in the fine print, however. These are not *confirmed* settings for the transmission, rather they are "potential community exposure settings."

13. Justin Hart (@justin_hart), "L.A. added another 130 locations…," Twitter, December 3, 2020, 12:51 a.m., https://twitter.com/justin_hart /status/1334374768418512897?s=20&t=h9A89QueQUdlQNvqTjx20A.

Chapter 2: You Must Trust "The Science™"! WRONG.

1. "Transcript: Dr. Anthony Fauci on 'Face the Nation,'" November 28, 2021, CBS News, November 28, 2021, https://www.cbsnews.com/news /transcript-dr-anthony-fauci-on-face-the-nation-november-28-2021/.

2. Michael Huling, "Anthony Fauci's Most Revealing Emails from FOIA Request," *American Conservative*, June 3, 2021, https://www.theamer icanconservative.com/state-of-the-union/anthony-faucis-most-revealing -emails-from-foia-request/.

3. Jay Battacharya (@DrJBattacharya), "The current generation of top public health leaders…," Twitter, April 17, 2022, 11:05 a.m., https://tw itter.com/DrJBhattacharya/status/1515707972798001156?s=20&t=1K wSPNIfYnj-wcBMVU8KIg.

4. Guardian News, "'Face Masks Are Our Best Defence,' Says CDC Director Redfield," YouTube, September 16, 2020, https://www.youtube.com/ watch?v=vOClXAg9nQU; Steven Nelson and Ebony Bowden, "CDC Director: Masks Are Better Defense against COVID-19 than Vaccine," *New York Post*, September 16, 2020, https://nypost.com/2020/09/16/cdc-director-masks-are-better-defense-against-covid-19-than-vaccine/; Matt Miller, "CDC Director Rochelle Walensky: No Concerns about Myocarditis with Nearly 5 Million Children Vaccinated," WFIN, December 10, 2021, https://wfin.com/abc-health/cdc-director-rochelle-walensky-no-concerns-about-myocarditis-with-nearly-5-million-children-vaccinated/; "Study Suggests COVID-19 Vaccines Do Not Reduce Fertility," National Institutes of Health, February 8, 2022, https://www.nih.gov/news-events/nih-research-matters/study-suggests-covid-19-vaccines-do-not-reduce-fertility.

5. Paul Sacca, "NIH Director Francis Collins Told Anthony Fauci There Needs to Be a 'Quick and Devastating' Takedown of Anti-Lockdown Declaration by 'Fringe' Harvard, Stanford, Oxford Epidemiologists: Emails," Blaze Media, December 18, 2021, https://www.theblaze.com/ news/fauci-email-francis-collins-great-barrington-declaration; "How Fauci and Collins Shut Down Covid Debate" (editorial), *Wall Street*

Journal, December 21, 2021, https://www.wsj.com/articles/fauci-collins
-emails-great-barrington-declaration-covid-pandemic-lockdown-11640
129116.

6. Jay Bhattacharya (@DrJBhattacharya), "Hospital staffing shortages are
at least in part...," Twitter, January 10, 2022, 11:42 p.m., https://twit
ter.com/DrJBhattacharya/status/1480761888963280898?s=20&t=ML
kyxWx6Osn3IxBV3SnY9A.

7. Nancy M. Baum, Peter D. Jacobson, and Susan D. Goold, "'Listen to
the People': Public Deliberation about Social Distancing Measures in a
Pandemic," *American Journal of Bioethics* 9, no. 11 (November 2009):
4, https://pubmed.ncbi.nlm.nih.gov/19882444/.

8. Ibid.

9. Ibid.

Chapter 3: The Pandemic Response Is Run by Intrepid Specialists! WRONG.

1. TRT World Now, "Coronavirus Outbreak: Interview with Anthony
Fauci, National Institutes of Health," YouTube, February 3, 2020,
https://www.youtube.com/watch?v=zepfDvHY-iE&t=183s.

2. Wendell Husebø, "Report: Anthony Fauci Said in Released Emails 'Drug
Store' Masks Are 'Not Really Effective,'" Breitbart, June 2, 2021, https://
www.breitbart.com/health/2021/06/02/report-anthony-fauci-said-relea
sed-emails-drug-store-masks-not-really-effective/.

3. Daniel Shields (@dwpshields), "March 1: 'Use an N95...," Twitter, June
5, 2021, 10:20 a.m., https://twitter.com/dwpshields/status/1401182023
008587778.

4. 60 Minutes, "March 2020: Dr. Anthony Fauci Talks with Dr. Jon
LaPook about Covid-19," YouTube, March 8, 2020, https://www.yout
ube.com/watch?v=PRa6t_e7dgI.

5. Miranda Devine, "Dr. Fauci Needs to Be Held Responsible for COVID-
19 Mistakes," *New York Post*, January 24, 2021, https://nypost.com/20
21/01/24/dr-fauci-needs-to-be-held-responsible-for-mistakes-devine/.

6. Personal communication with Scott Atlas.
7. Steven Nelson and Ebony Bowden, "CDC Director: Masks Are Better Defense against COVID-19 Than Vaccine," *New York Post*, September 16, 2020, https://nypost.com/2020/09/16/cdc-director-masks-are-better -defense-against-covid-19-than-vaccine/.

Chapter 4: Fauci's Gain-of-Function Research Is a Conspiracy Theory! WRONG.

1. The timeline for the emergence of SARS-CoV-2 is full of mystery. Here's a brief rundown of what transpired. This timeline follows the story from China. A subsequent timeline outlines the gain-of-function research funded by the U.S. National Institutes of Health.

   In 2012 six miners in China were hospitalized with an outbreak of severe, unexplained pneumonia.

   In 2016 a Chinese researcher published claims that some of the miners had SARS antibodies and revealed that the event occurred in the village of Danaoshan.

   China blocks roads and information about the copper mine and censors any reports related to the illnesses.

   Numerous research groups conduct genome studies to examine the newfound SARS incident. These projects and their findings are kept in secrecy.

   In 2017 a paper by Dr. Zhengli with the intent to produce research is made public. The paper was titled: "Study on the Evolutionary Mechanism of Bat SARS-Like Coronavirus Adapted to Host Receptor Molecules and the Risk of Cross-Species Infection."

   In 2018 research conducted on SARS-related coronaviruses identifies the ACE2 receptor as a leading candidate for triggering an illness.

   Also in 2018 the Chinese Academy of Sciences (CAS) initiated a project to develop vaccines based on previously published bat coronavirus research.

In 2019 the Wuhan Institute of Virology starts upgrades for critical biosafety examinations.

Odd patents are issued to the Wuhan lab for high-grade biosafety laboratory disinfectant and treatment of wounds from lab accidents.

Wuhan published information indicating that they were conducting experiments with rabbits, rats, mutant mice, ferrets, and bats for experimental purposes.

Also in 2019, SARS-CoV-2 is identified by Chinese officials at a wet market in Wuhan.

Shortly thereafter, the lead epidemiologist for the team investigating the outbreak issues a directive not to "provide other institutions and individuals with information related to Covid-19 epidemic on their own including data, biological specimens, pathogens, culture etc."

Also important is a timeline running concurrently with the research and subsequent outbreak in Wuhan. This timeline details the shady and dangerous "gain of function" research approved by the NIH and Dr. Fauci and promoted in conjunction with the Wuhan Institute through various partners of the United States.

1999: The Department of Health and Human Services (HHS) funds research amplifying the infectious-character coronaviruses, known as gain of function.

2000: Researcher Ralph Baric submits a patent reverse engineering SARS-CoV.

2002–2006: Scientists in the United States and China file patents for combining the DNA of coronaviruses with HIV and other diseases.

2011: Scientists raise alarms about gain-of-function research after labs in Wisconsin and the Netherlands mutate a lethal strain of the H5N1 avian flu.

2013: MERS outbreak in the Middle East. This same year, Baric and Chinese scientists isolate three coronaviruses from bats examining spike protein behaviors.

2014: CDC accidentally exposes workers to anthrax and ships deadly virus of smallpox. Obama administration halts gain-of-function research.

2015: Baric and Chinese researcher Dr. Zhengli announce they have "reengineered HKU4 spike aiming to build its capacity to mediate viral entry into human cells."

2017: The gain-of-function research ban is lifted.

2018: The research by Dr. Zhengli is published (later taken down by Chinese officials).

Summer 2019: Researchers from Wuhan request that their genome additions to the NIH genome databank be deleted. NIH complies.

December 2019: SARS-CoV-2 outbreak

These two timelines merge to tell a story of researchers playing with fire and perhaps, accidentally setting the world alight as a result. See Derrick Bryson Taylor, "A Timeline of the Coronavirus Pandemic," *New York Times*, March 17, 2021, https://www.nytimes.com/article/coronavirus-timeline.html; Katherine Eban, "The Lab-Leak Theory: Inside the Fight to Uncover COVID-19's Origins," *Vanity Fair*, June 3, 2021, https://www.vanityfair.com/news/2021/06/the-lab-leak-theory-inside-the-fight-to-uncover-covid-19s-origins; Monali C. Rahalkar and Rahul A. Bahulikar, "Lethal Pneumonia Cases in Mojiang Miners (2012) and the Mineshaft Could Provide Important Clues to the Origin of SARS-CoV-2," *Frontiers in Public Health* 8, no. 581569 (October 20, 2020), https://www.frontiersin.org/articles/10.3389/fpubh.2020.581569/full; Glenn Kessler, "Timeline: How the Wuhan Lab-Leak Theory Suddenly Became Credible," *Washington Post*, May 25, 2021, https://www.washingtonpost.com/politics/2021/05/25/timeline-how-wuhan-lab-leak-theory-suddenly-became-credible/; Jenny Lei Ravelo and Sara Jerving, "COVID-19 in 2021—a Timeline of the Coronavirus Outbreak," Devex, January 20, 2022, https://www.devex.com/news/covid-19-in-2021-a-timeline-of-the-coronavirus-outbreak-102417; Jamie Metzl, "Origins of SARS-CoV-2," Jamie Metzl, June 22, 2022, https://jamiemetzl.com/origins-of-sars-cov-2/.

2. Jon Cohen, "Mining Coronavirus Genomes for Clues to the Outbreak's Origins," *Science*, January 31, 2020, https://www.science.org/content /article/mining-coronavirus-genomes-clues-outbreak-s-origins.

3. Joe Concha, "Media Continues to Lionize Anthony Fauci, despite His Damning Emails," *The Hill*, June 5, 2021, https://thehill.com/opinion/ healthcare/556891-media-continues-to-lionize-anthony-fauci-despite -his-damning-emails/; Samuel Chamberlain, "Sen. Paul: Fauci Emails Prove He Knew of Wuhan Gain-of-Function Research," *New York Post*, June 3, 2021, https://nypost.com/2021/06/03/fauci-emails-prove-he-kn ew-of-wuhan-research-sen-paul/; Andrew Chapados, "Fauci Emails Show Top Doc Was Concerned about 'Gain of Function' Research as Early as Jan. 2020," RebelNews, June 2, 2021, https://www.rebelnews .com/fauci_emails_gain_of_function_research_coronavirus.

Chapter 5: Covid Spreads Only by Droplets in the Breath! WRONG.

1. CNN (@CNN), "'I would be terrified . . . ,'" Twitter, May 14, 2020, 6:41 p.m., https://twitter.com/CNN/status/1261063993730326530?s=20& t=MLkyxWx6Osn3IxBV3SnY9A.

2. KUSI News, "Wooten: Assume everyone has COVID-19," Facebook, August 19, 2020, 6:30 p.m., https://www.facebook.com/watch/?v=339 609623892702.

Chapter 6: Everyone Is at Serious Risk from Covid! WRONG.

1. Jonathan Rothwell, "U.S. Adults' Estimates of COVID-19 Hospitalization Risk," Gallup, September 27, 2021, https://news.gallup.com/opinion /gallup/354938/adults-estimates-covid-hospitalization-risk.aspx.

2. Cathrine Axfors and John P. A. Ioannidis, "Infection Fatality Rate of COVID-19 in Community-Dwelling Populations with Emphasis on the Elderly: An Overview," medRxiv, July 13, 2021, https://www.medrxiv .org/content/10.1101/2021.07.08.21260210v1.full.pdf.

3. Compare ages at 20 years apart:

    20 years old: 268 Covid deaths and 9,670 other deaths

    40 years old: 2,812 Covid deaths and 28,061 other deaths

    60 years old: 15,375 Covid deaths and 113,767 other deaths

    80 years old: 25,827 Covid deaths and 198,239 other deaths

    "Provisional COVID-19 Death Counts by Age in Years, 2020–2022," Centers for Disease Control and Prevention, June 29, 2022, https://data .cdc.gov/NCHS/Provisional-COVID-19-Death-Counts-by-Age-in-Years -/3apk-4u4f.

4. "Provisional COVID-19 Death Counts by Sex and Age," Centers for Disease Control and Prevention, June 29, 2022, https://data.cdc.gov/NC HS/Provisional-COVID-19-Deaths-by-Sex-and-Age/9bhg-hcku.

5. Here are some comparisons:

    19 years old: 1 in 37,000 odds of dying. Similar to the odds of dying from a sharp object

    20 to 29 years old: 1 in 7000 odds of dying. Similar to the odds of dying from sunstroke

    30 to 39 years old: 1 in 3225 odds of dying. Similar to the odds of dying from choking on food

    40 to 49 years old: 1 in 1200 odds of dying. Similar to the odds of dying from drowning

    50 to 59 years old: 1 in 350 odds of dying. Similar to the odds of dying in a pedestrian accident

    60 to 69 years old: 1 in 150 odds of dying. Similar to the odds of dying in a car crash

    70+ years old: 1 in 41 odds of dying. Similar to the odds of dying of a chronic respiratory disease

    For Covid stats, see "Provisional COVID-19 Death Counts by Sex and Age"; for comparable risks, see "Facts + Statistics: Morality Risk," Insurance Information Institute, 2022, https://www.iii.org/fact-statistic/ facts-statistics-mortality-risk.

6. Berkeley Lovelace Jr. and Noah Higgins-Dunn, "WHO Says Coronavirus Death Rate Is 3.4% Globally, Higher than Previously Thought," CNBC, March 3, 2020, https://www.cnbc.com/2020/03/03 /who-says-coronavirus-death-rate-is-3point4percent-globally-higher-th an-previously-thought.html.

7. Jacob Sullum, "Is a 1% Case Fatality Rate for COVID-19 Bad News or Good News?," *Reason*, March 12, 2020, https://reason.com/2020/03 /12/is-a-1-case-fatality-rate-for-covid-19-bad-news-or-good-news/.

8. Justin Hart (@justin_hart), "Setting expectations for vaccine watchers....," Twitter, October 8, 2020, 5:02 p.m., https://twitter.com/ justin_hart/status/1314310202129174529?s=20&t=TSdBmLIfjJXqA5E SoFJXow; "Estimated Flu-Related Illnesses, Medical Visits, Hospitalizations, and Deaths in the United States—2017–2018 Flu Season," Centers for Disease Control and Prevention, September 30, 2021, https://www.cdc.gov/flu/about/burden/2017-2018.htm.

9. Justin Hart (@justin_hart), "One line represents cumulative U.S. C19 deaths . . . ," Twitter, March 31, 2022, 5:39 p.m., https://twitter.com/ justin_hart/status/1509646543426531330?s=20&t=TSdBmLIfjJXqA5E SoFJXow; "NYTimes/Covid-19-Data," GitHub, 2022, https://github. com/nytimes/covid-19-data.

10. What *do* people die of? The CDC itemizes the underlying cause of death into codes known as ICD-10 codes. Every so often the CDC puts out a dataset titled "Weekly Provisional Counts of Deaths by State and Select Causes." They typically have only published data for 2020–2021, but if you search hard enough, you can get it back to 2014. The select causes are these:

    Alzheimer disease (G30)
    COVID-19 (U071, Multiple Cause of Death)
    COVID-19 (U071, Underlying Cause of Death)
    Cerebrovascular diseases (I60-I69)
    Chronic lower respiratory diseases (J40-J47)
    Diabetes mellitus (E10-E14)

Diseases of heart (I00-I09, I11, I13, I20-I51)

Influenza and pneumonia (J09-J18)

Malignant neoplasms (C00-C97)

Nephritis, nephrotic syndrome, and nephrosis (N00-N07, N17-N19, N25-N27)

Other diseases of respiratory system (J00-J06, J30-J39, J67, J70-J98)

Septicemia (A40-A41)

Symptoms, signs, and abnormal clinical and laboratory findings, not elsewhere classified (R00-R99)

These categories are from "AH Monthly Provisional Counts of Deaths by Age Group and HHS Region for Select Causes of Death, 2019–2021," Centers for Disease Control and Prevention, April 1, 2021, https://data.cdc.gov/NCHS/AH-Monthly-Provisional-Counts-of-Deaths-by-Age-Gro/ezfr-g6hf.

It's this last one that I'm interested in. In May 2020 we did some investigating into signs that Covid might have been here previously. We examined data to show that the rise in deaths attributed to this category (R00-R99) had risen considerably. In other words, there were a whole bunch of deaths before Covid was said to have arrived that the CDC couldn't really categorize.

Is it possible that COVID-19 had been with us much earlier than we anticipated? What's more, as we look over the range of potential causes of deaths, we note that there are many crossovers with deaths of COVID-19. Alzheimer deaths hit a record high in 2020 and waned a bit in 2021. What does this indicate? Were these Alzheimer/Covid deaths already nearing the threshold of this mortal existence? Should that minimize our fears and inform our policies on COVID-19, knowing that a good portion of deaths are possibly *incidental* in the big net theory?

Chapter 7: If You Die *with* Covid, Then You Die *from* Covid! WRONG.

1. Dag Gano, "Kary Mullis on Fauci," YouTube, December 8, 2020, https://patriotnet.com/videos/806/1838/kary-mullis-on-fauci.

2. Ibid.

3. Tim Meads, "After CDC's Rochelle Walensky Admits COVID-19 PCR Tests Have a Major Flaw, Conservatives Demand Answers," Daily Wire+, December 29, 2021, https://www.dailywire.com/news/after-cdcs-rochelle-walensky-admits-covid-19-pcr-tests-has-a-major-flaw-conservatives-demand-answers.

4. David Zweig, "Our Most Reliable Pandemic Number Is Losing Meaning," *The Atlantic*, September 13, 2021, https://www.theatlantic.com/health/archive/2021/09/covid-hospitalization-numbers-can-be-misleading/620062/; Bruce Golding, "Over 40% of NYC's COVID-Infected Hospital Patients Admitted for Other Reasons," *New York Post*, January 7, 2022, https://nypost.com/2022/01/07/many-nyc-patients-hospitalized-with-covid-admitted-for-other-reasons/.

5. "Reporting COVID Deaths," Oregon Health Authority, https://www.oregon.gov/oha/PH/BIRTHDEATHCERTIFICATES/VITALSTATISTICS/DEATH/Pages/reporting-covid-deaths.aspx; "Department of Public Health Updates COVID-19 Death Definition," Mass.gov, March 10, 2022, https://www.mass.gov/news/department-of-public-health-updates-covid-19-death-definition; "Coronavirus Disease 2019," County of Los Angeles Public Health, http://publichealth.lacounty.gov/acd/ncorona2019/reporting.htm.

6. Sara G. Murray, Rhiannon Croci, and Robert M. Wachter, "Is a Patient Hospitalized 'with' Covid or 'for' Covid? Is Can Be Hard to Tell," *Washington Post*, January 7, 2022, https://www.washingtonpost.com/outlook/2022/01/07/hospitalization-covid-statistics-incidental/.

7. Bethania Palma, "Are Doctors and Hospitals Paid More for COVID-19 Patients?," Snopes, April 17, 2020, https://www.snopes.com/fact-check/medicare-hospitals-covid-patients/; "Critical Access and Small, Rural

Hospitals to Receive Cares Act Funds," Illinois Critical Access Hospital Network, April 2, 2020, https://icahn.org/news/critical-access-and-small-rural-hospitals-to-receive-cares-act-funds/; "Critical Access Hospitals (CAHs)," Rural Health Information Hub, September 3, 2021, https://www.ruralhealthinfo.org/topics/critical-access-hospitals.

8. Jen Christensen, "How the Pandemic Killed a Record Number of Rural Hospitals," CNN Health, July 31, 2021, https://www.cnn.com/2021/07/31/health/rural-hospital-closures-pandemic/index.html.

9. Danielle Ofri, "The Public Has Been Forgiving. But Hospitals Got Some Things Wrong," *New York Times*, May 22, 2020, https://www.nytimes.com/2020/05/22/opinion/sunday/coronavirus-medical-errors-hospitals.html.

10. "CDC Overreported COVID-19 Deaths by More than 70,000," Daily Wire+, March 23, 2022, https://www.dailywire.com/news/cdc-overreported-covid-19-deaths-by-more-than-70000.

11. Gano, "Kary Mullis on Fauci."

12. Jon Kamp, Stephanie Stamm, and Elliot Bentley, "U.S. Surpasses One Million Covid-19 Deaths," *Wall Street Journal*, May 16, 2022, https://www.wsj.com/articles/u-s-nears-one-million-covid-19-deaths-11650838998.

13. For instance, back in the summer of 2020, our Team Reality colleagues Jennifer and Len Cabrera got the opportunity to review about seven hundred redacted COVID-19 death certificates. As a brief explanation, there are two parts to a death certificate:

"The certificate has a clear 'manner of death' by category (e.g., natural, homicide, accident, etc.). PART 1 should describe the chain of events that directly caused the death. Line *a* should be the immediate cause of death, followed by the events that result from the underlying cause, which is listed last." They continue: "Line *a* is considered the 'mechanism of death,' but the CDC does not require listing a 'terminal event' such as cardiac or respiratory arrest. PART 2 lists other significant contributing diseases or conditions that did not result in the underlying cause of death."

From their analysis (published on Rational Ground and their local news site, AlachuaChronicle.com) they deemed a full third of the death certificates "interesting"—that is, certificates with causes of death that were possible frauds. Jennifer Cabrera and Len Cabrera, "Florida Death Certificate Review Raises Questions about Official Number of COVID-19 Deaths," Rational Ground, November 11, 2020, https://rationalground.com/florida-death-certificate-review-raises-questions-about-official-number-of-covid-19-deaths/; Jennifer Cabrera and Len Cabrera, "Death Certificate Review Raises Questions about Official Number of COVID-19 Deaths," Alachua Chronicle, October 30, 2020, https://alachuachronicle.com/death-certificate-review-raises-questions-about-official-number-of-covid-19-deaths/.

14. Team Reality colleagues Jennifer and Len Cabrera reviewed about seven hundred redacted COVID-19 death certificates from summer 2020. Here are some of the more notable deaths they recorded for your review. The format here is age, sex, and then a description of the listing of the causes of death.

   84M, PART 1: a. Cerebrovascular accident, b. atherosclerosis, PART 2: COVID-19 pneumonia

   85M, PART 1: a. Ischemic cardiomyopathy, PART 2: Chronic kidney disease, COVID-19

   57M, PART 1: a. Coronary artery disease, PART 2: asymptomatic COVID-19 positive swab

   88M, PART 1: a. Failure to thrive, b. dementia, c. type II diabetes, PART 2: COVID-19 positive

   79F, PART 1: a. renal cancer—4 months, PART 2: COVID-19

   56F, PART 1: a. complications of paraplegia (non-traumatic), PART 2: Chronic obstructive pulmonary disease, diabetes mellitus, COVID-19

   77F, Accident, PART 1: a. exacerbation of COVID-19 pneumonia, b. prolonged bed rest, c. left femoral neck and pelvic fracture, d. fall, PART 2: fall from standing height

96M, PART 1: a. hypertensive cardiovascular disease, PART 2: renal insufficiency, anemia, COVID-19

59M, PART 1: a. cardiorespiratory arrest, b. failure to thrive, c. developmental delay, PART 2: COVID-19, urosepsis

90F, PART 1: a. cardiopulmonary arrest 2nd to arrhythmia, b. failure to thrive, c. recovered from COVID-19, PART 2: dementia, HTN, hypothyroid

98F, PART 1: a. Cerebral atherosclerosis, b. vascular dementia without, c. behavioral disturbances, d. COVID-19 positive, PART 2: chronic fatigue, respiratory distress

74F, Accident, PART 1: a. COVID-19 infection & bronchopulmonary aspergillosis complicating sequelae of blunt force injury of right, PART 2: diabetes, hypertension, cardiovascular disease, obesity

84F, PART 1: a. Alzheimer's, PART 2: COVID-19 disease

88M, PART 1: a. cancer of larynx, PART 2: COVID-19 infection

85F, PART 1: a. Arteriosclerotic CV disease, PART 2: Atrial fibrillation, COVID-19

41M, PART 1: a. Cardiac arrest—immediate b. Respiratory failure, acute on [sic] chronic—days c. Pulmonary artery hypertension—years d. Sarcoidosis—years, PART 2: COVID-19

69M, PART 1: a. Multiple ischemic strokes, PART 2: Chronic renal failure, recent COVID-19 pneu, dementia

70M, PART 1: a. Natural causes—years, PART 2: Neurocognitive (congenital developmental) delay, COVID-19 infection, recurrent aspiration pneumonia

60M, PART 1: a. Septic shock—days b. E Coli Bacterium-UTI c. GI bleed—acute blood loss anemia-esophageal necrosis d. acute hypoxemic respiratory failure, PART 2: Hypertension, HX of COVID

88F, PART 1: a. Complications of dementia, PART 2: Atrial fibrillation, arteriosclerotic cardiovascular disease, COVID-19

79F, PART 1: a. Coronary artery disease—years, PART 2: COVID-19, myeloproliferative disorder, diabetes, Parkinson's

83F, Accident, PART 1: a. Complications of COVID-19—NS, PART 2: Traumatic brain injury, failure to thrive, atherosclerotic and hypertensive cardiovascular disease, urinary tract infection

87F, PART 1: a. Senile degeneration of brain, PART 2: Complications related to COVID-19 infection

98F, PART 1: a. End stage dementia b. Adult failure to thrive c. Positive COVID-19, PART 2: blank

64M, PART 1: a. Acute heart failure b. Chronic systolic heart failure c. Ischemic cardiomyopathy d. A. Fib, hypertension, HLD, PART 2: COVID-19

72M, PART 1: a. Parkinson's disease, PART 2: Hypertension, history of COVID-19 and deep vein thrombosis in July

89M, PART 1: a. Cardiorespiratory arrest b. Failure to thrive c. Arteriosclerosis cardiovascular disease, PART 2: COVID-19

82F, PART 1: a. Unknown b. Failure to thrive, depression—7 days c. Exposure to COVID-19, cough and shortness of breath—14 days d. Dementia, hypothyroidism, atrial fibrillation, bronchospasm, congestive heart failure—years, PART 2: History of refusing medications and food for at least 7 days, refusal to go to the emergency room

77M, PART 1: a. Stage 4 small cell carcinoma of the lung, PART 2: COPD, COVID-19 pneumonia, hypertension

61M, PART 1: a. Metastasis to liver of unknown origin b. Adenocarcinoma c. COVID-19 d. Severe protein-calorie malnutrition, PART 2: blank

69F, PART 1: a. Glioblastoma—months, PART 2: COVID-19 pneu

78F, PART 1: a. End stage Parkinson's disease, PART 2: COVID-19 pneu, HTN, CAD

83M, PART 1: a. Dementia b. Parkinson's c. B Cell chronic lymphocytic leukemia d. CKD-III, PART 2: COVID-19

81F, PART 1: a. Small bowel obstruction—weeks, PART 2: CHF, renal failure, dementia, COVID-19

62M, PART 1: a. Severe sepsis due to obstructive pneumonia—5 days b. right lung mass, likely cancer—60 days, PART 2: Acute renal failure, brain metastasis, COVID-19 infection

90F, PART 1: a. complications of dementia, PART 2: Arteriosclerotic cardiovascular disease, COVID-19

76M, PART 1: a. Cardiorespiratory arrest b. End stage renal disease in hemodialysis c. insulin dependent diabetes mellitus, PART 2: Cerebrovascular accident, HTN, hyperlipidemia schizophrenia necrotic sacululcar [sic] COVID-19 infection

72M, PART 1: a. Esophageal adenocarcinoma with lung and liver metastases, PART 2: COVID-19 pneumonia

57M, PART 1: a. Myocardial infarction, PART 2: COVID-19 infection

75M, PART 1: a. End stage ALS, PART 2: Respiratory failure secondary to COVID-19

94F, PART 1: a. Arteriosclerotic cardiovascular disease, PART 2: Hypertension, dementia, COVID-19

90F, PART 1: a. Cerebrovascular accident b. Atrial fibrillation, PART 2: COVID (6/2020)

87M, PART 1: a. Cardiorespiratory arrest b. dilated cardiomyopathy c. aortic insufficiency/secondary to AV block d. COPD, PART 2: Parkinson's, vascular dementia, duodenal ulcer, H/O COVID+

92F, PART 1: a. Sequelae of femoral neck fracture b. Blunt impact to extremity, PART 2: Asymptomatic COVID-19 infection, hypertensive heart disease

65M, PART 1: a. Complications of hepatocellular carcinoma, PART 2: Obesity, COPD, COVID-19, hypertension

69F, PART 1: a. Complications of urinary tract infection, PART 2: Chronic ethanolism, COVID-19, hypertension, diabetes mellitus

92F, PART 1: a. Sepsis b. Multidrug resistant bacteremia, PART 2: Decubital wound, COVID-19, dementia, chronic kidney disease stage III, hypertension, diabetes mellitus type II, hyperlipidemia

94M, PART 1: a. Multiple diseases of the elderly, PART 2: Cerebrovascular disease, vascular dementia, hypertension, chronic lymphocytic leukemia, atrial fibrillation, COVID positivity

88M, PART 1: a. Multiple diseases of the elderly, PART 2: Cerebrovascular disease with previous strokes, vascular dementia, COVID-19 positivity, hypertension

61M, PART 1: a. Hepatocellular carcinoma, Hepatitis C, PART 2: COVID-19, non-small cell lung cancer, cirrhosis

97F, Accident, PART 1: a. Complications of right intertrochanteric femur fracture, PART 2: Hypertensive and arteriosclerotic cardiovascular disease with congestive heart failure, complications of COVID-19

52F, PART 1: a. Liver failure b. Metastatic disease c. Breast cancer, PART 2: Coagulopathy, septic shock, COVID-19

80M, PART 1: a. Dementia b. Cerebrovascular disease c. COPD d. Coronary artery disease, PART 2: C19+

90M, PART 1: a. Octogenarian natural causes b. S/P C19, PART 2: blank

97M, PART 1: a. Complications of dementia, PART 2: CKD, COVID-19, Protein calorie malnutrition, Arteriosclerotic cardiovascular disease

60F, PART 1: a. Intracranial bleed b. End stage liver disease, PART 2: Pneu, COVID-19 positive history, hypertension, cirrhosis, anemia

89F, Accident, PART 1: a. Complications of hip fracture, PART 2: Cerebrovascular accident, Arteriosclerotic and hypertensive cardiovascular disease, dementia, COVID-19

91F, PART 1: a. Left hip ORIF repair b. COVID + history c. CABG X 4 vessels d. Heart failure, PART 2: COPD

You can pick out a few, but you can see from those last two the wide measures that were used to log Covid deaths. Eighty-nine-year-old woman fractured her hip and had a history of heart disease and dementia. Conclusion: Covid death. Ninety-one-year-old female had some heart issues and passed away while having a hip repair. Previous history of Covid. Conclusion: Covid death.

The Cabrera's full analysis is available on Rational Ground and their local news site AlachuaChronicle.com. Jennifer Cabrera and Len Cabrera, "Florida Death Certificate Review Raises Questions about Official Number of COVID-19 Deaths," Rational Ground, November 11, 2020, https://rationalground.com/florida-death-certificate-review-raises-quest ions-about-official-number-of-covid-19-deaths/; Jennifer Cabrera and Lend Cabrera, "Death Certificate Review Raises Questions about Official Number of COVID-19 Deaths," Alachua Chronicle, October 30, 2020, https://alachuachronicle.com/death-certificate-review-raises-questions-ab out-official-number-of-covid-19-deaths/.

15. "CDC Reports Fewer Covid-19 Pediatric Deaths after Data Correction," Reuters, March 18, 2022, https://www.reuters.com/business/healthcare -pharmaceuticals/cdc-reports-fewer-covid-19-pediatric-deaths-after-da ta-correction-2022-03-18/.

16. In their vaunted Case Surveillance File, the CDC has specific measures for each case that is logged in the massive data file. They denote the type of date on record: 1) a confirmed date for the onset of illness; 2) a date for a positive specimen taken from the case; or 3) a reported date, when the case was logged. Ideally, that is the desired pecking order of data we want attached to each case.

For example, if there is an onset-of-illness date, then that implies an actual person-to-person interview with a positive case. If we don't have that, the date for a positive case result is excellent. As a last resort, if we don't have the date when the person tested positive, it defaults to when the case was entered in the system. Additionally, the data file denotes whether it is a lab-confirmed case or a probable case.

In terms of traditional virus measurements, we like to have the earliest date and lab-confirmed case, and if the case turns into death, it would be great to see a hospitalization status. Here's a quick cascade of the stats from the CDC as of June 2022:

856,278 deaths with COVID-19

577,575 deaths with a clinical date

530,077 deaths with a lab-confirmed positive test

329,162 deaths with a confirmed hospitalization

"COVID-19 Case Surveillance Public Use Data," Centers for Disease Control and Prevention, June 9, 2022, https://data.cdc.gov/Case-Surveil lance/COVID-19-Case-Surveillance-Public-Use-Data/vbim-akqf.

If we are to use consistent approaches outlined by the CDC in assessing the *burdens* of COVID-19, we would have to conclude that there are only 277,000 deaths in their system. The rest are questionable, to say the least. The data are very, very bad.

17. Apoorva Mandavilli, "The C.D.C. Isn't Publishing Large Portions of the Covid Data It Collects," *New York Times*, February 20, 2022, https://www.nytimes.com/2022/02/20/health/covid-cdc-data.html.

18. Lauren Brownlie, "Covid Data Will Not Be Published over Concerns It's Misrepresented by Anti-Vaxxers," *Glasgow Times*, February 17, 2022, https://www.glasgowtimes.co.uk/news/19931641.covid-data-wi ll-not-published-concerns-misrepresented-anti-vaxxers/.

19. Clayton Cobb, "How Prominent Public Health Agencies Are Skewing Vaccine Effectiveness Statistics in the US—#Denominatorgate," Blaze Media, February 21, 2022, https://www.theblaze.com/news/denomina torgate-how-public-health-agencies-are-skewing-the-statistics-on-vacci ne-effectiveness.

20. Our colleague Clayton Cobb (@HOLD2LLC on Twitter) demonstrated in data procured from New York State authorities that numerous factors reduce the difference of 1000 percent close to two times decreased risk. As of this writing that difference is practically zero in many locations. Vaccine efficacy wanes and vaccine data is unreliable, leading to huge policy blunders around mandates. Cobb, "How Prominent Public Health Agencies."

21. "COVID-19 Vaccination Coverage and Vaccine Confidence among Adults," Centers for Disease Control and Prevention, https://www.cdc.gov/vaccines/imz-managers/coverage/covidvaxview/interactive/adults.html; "COVID-19 Vaccination and Case Trends by Age Group, United

States," Centers for Disease Control and Prevention, https://data.cdc.gov/Vaccinations/COVID-19-Vaccination-and-Case-Trends-by-Age-Group-/gxj9-t96f.

22. "Provisional COVID-19 Death Counts by Age in Years, 2020–2022," Centers for Disease Control and Prevention, June 29, 2022, https://data.cdc.gov/NCHS/Provisional-COVID-19-Death-Counts-by-Age-in-Years-/3apk-4u4f.

23. About 14 percent of all those surveyed by the CDC answered affirmative to this query: "Probably or Definitely Will Not Get Vaccinated." If you extrapolate populations for the categories above based on the most recent surveys, it breaks down this way for the adamantly hesitant:

Approximately five million "hesitant" eighteen-to-twenty-nine-year-olds

Eight million thirty-year-olds

Sixteen million forty-to-sixty-five-year-olds

Six million others

That's about thirty-four million hesitant across the board and another nineteen million who plan to get or will probably get the vaccine.

There are nearly *two hundred million* adults (18+) in the United States under the age of sixty-five. About *one hundred forty thousand* Covid deaths have occurred in that age range. "COVID-19 Vaccination Coverage and Vaccine Confidence among Adults," Centers for Disease Control and Prevention, September 23, 2021, https://www.cdc.gov/vaccines/imz-managers/coverage/covidvaxview/interactive/adults.html.

Chapter 8: If You Don't Wear a Mask, You're Killing Grandma! WRONG.

1. Robby Soave, "CNN's Leana Wen: 'Cloth Masks Are Little More than Facial Decorations,'" *Reason*, December 21, 2021, https://reason.com/2021/12/21/leana-wen-cloth-mask-facial-decorations-covid-cdc-guidance/.

2. Michael Klompas et al., "Universal Masking in Hospitals in the Covid-19 Era," *New England Journal of Medicine* 382, no. 63 (May 21, 2020), https://www.nejm.org/doi/full/10.1056/nejmp2006372.

3. Andre Neveling, "Did Michael Jackson 'Predict' Covid-19? How MJ's Face Masks, Daughter Paris, a Finding Neverland Sequel and a Homeless Statue Continue to Make Headlines 11 Years after the King of Pop's Death," *South China Morning Post*, February 23, 2021, https://www.scmp.com/magazines/style/celebrity/article/3122627/did-michael-jackson-predict-covid-19-how-mjs-face-masks.

4. "Michael Jackson Predicted Coronavirus Type Pandemic," Yahoo! News, March 25, 2020, https://nz.news.yahoo.com/michael-jackson-predicted-coronavirus-type-150658401.html.

5. Yes, strippers. The schools and gyms had to close, but it was determined that these establishments of repute—the vaunted American stripper bars—could keep their doors open. The strippers, of course, are carefully monitored, and all of them have to wear masks. California stripper Brittany told Reuters in May 2021 that an hour of that four-hour shift was spent just waiting for customers and she earned $150, less than a third of what she would have made pre-pandemic. "Strippers Are Back on the Job but COVID Rules Are Hurting Their Pay," Reuters, May 18, 2021, https://www.reuters.com/world/us/strippers-are-back-job-covid-rules-are-hurting-their-pay-2021-05-18/.

    With all of the boisterous interactions at these strip clubs, it was clear that masking impacted business and frankly—as everyone knew—wasn't really helping with the spread of the disease—Covid or otherwise.

Chapter 9: Masks Are Imperfect but Keep Covid in Check! WRONG.

1. A fuller list includes:

    Streptococcus pneumoniae (pneumonia)

    Mycobacterium tuberculosis (tuberculosis)

    Neisseria meningitidis (meningitis, sepsis)

Acanthamoeba polyphaga (keratitis and granulomatous amebic encephalitis)

Acinetobacter baumanni (pneumonia, blood stream infections, meningitis, UTIs—resistant to antibiotics)

Escherichia coli (food poisoning)

Borrelia burgdorferi (causes Lyme disease)

Corynebacterium diphtheriae (diphtheria)

Legionella pneumophila (Legionnaires' disease)

Staphylococcus pyogenes serotype M3 (severe infections—high morbidity rates)

Staphylococcus aureus (meningitis, sepsis)

This list is from Jennifer Cabrera, "Dangerous Pathogens Found on Children's Face Masks," Rational Ground, June 16, 2021, https://rationalground.com/dangerous-pathogens-found-on-childrens-face-masks/.

2. Cabrera, "Dangerous Pathogens Found on Children's Face Masks."

3. Here are some excerpts Rational Ground gathered from various published papers to support these assertions:

"Our data indicate that children are at far greater risk of critical illness from influenza than from COVID-19." (JAMA Network)

"Children and young people remain at low risk from COVID-19 mortality." (OSF PrePrint)

"…children are not the main drivers of SARS-CoV-2 transmission." (CMAJ Group)

Children rarely transmit infection to others and more frequently have an asymptomatic or mild course compared to adults. (Journal of Medical Virology)

Asymptomatic spread in long-exposure, household settings was less than 1%. (JAMA Network)

"…could not provide evidence for a relevant asymptomatic spread…in childcare facilities…in a low nor a high prevalence setting." (medRxiv)

"For adults living with children there is no evidence of an increased risk of severe COVID outcomes" (medRxiv)

Increased household exposure to kids was associated w/ a smaller risk of testing positive or hospitalization w/ Covid (medRxiv)

"...we did not note any association between mask use and risk..." (The Lancet)

"Evidence regarding the effectiveness of non-medical face masks for the prevention of COVID-19 is scarce." (ECDC)

"...people must not touch their masks, must change their single-use masks frequently or wash them regularly..." (BMJ)

The effectiveness of high-grade masks for flu was linked to correct usage. (NIH)

Children have a lower tolerance to wearing masks and may fail to use them properly. (ECDC)

"...household use of face masks is associated with low adherence and is ineffective for controlling seasonal respiratory disease." (EID)

"...it's difficult for some autistic people to wear masks because of sensitivity issues," (OAR)

Deaf and Disabled children can feel isolated from other children and adults who are wearing masks. (The Guardian)

"Extended mask-wearing by the general population could lead to relevant effects and consequences in many medical fields." (MDPI)

"Psychosocial, biological, and immunological risks for children and pupils..." (BMJ)

School masks: face coverings could damage children's speech development, warn scientists. (The Telegraph)

"...wearing masks throughout the day can hinder language and socio-emotional development, particularly for younger children." (AAP)

A database tracking mask mandates has seen no clear benefit to masking children (Qualtrics Dashboard)

"...the data shows that districts' face covering policies do not impact the spread of the virus," (FL Education Board)

Delta does not seem to change the game. No difference in risk of hospitalization between Delta variant and Alpha (medRxiv)

The viral dynamics of the Delta variant are similar to those of Alpha. (medRxiv)

Studies in favor of school masking have been extremely flawed. The North Carolina study was done without a control group. (WSJ)

This list is from Justin Hart, "Masking Children Is an Ineffective Policy and Not Supported by Research or Data," Rational Ground (Substack), September 30, 2021, https://covidreason.substack.com/p/masking-children-is-an-ineffective.

4. "Where People around the World Find Meaning in Life," Pew Research Center, November 18, 2021, https://www.pewresearch.org/global/interactives/meaning-in-life/data/united-states.

5. Dan Rather (@DanRather), "Mask not what your country . . . ," Twitter, October 23, 2020, 11:20 p.m., https://twitter.com/DanRather/status/1319841263563067392?s=20&t=yo1xEqiydTkwROiuIqHZdQ.

6. One mom put a virtuous spin on Elf on a Shelf during Christmas. The note from the elf reads: "I am here for a visit. Santa said I could. I've been tested for Covid. The test came back good. This virus is awful, and even blue, but with me around, oh the fun things we will do. Wash your hands and keep your distance so Santa can see you're always consistent."

The elf accompanies the letter in person, fully masked, inside a tightly closed jar, with a bottle of hand-sanitizer to boot. Kish (fringe) (@kishkitsch), "The number of local fb moms…," Twitter, December 1, 2020, 12:10 p.m., https://twitter.com/kishkitsch/status/1333820841096851460?s=20&t=Xb6Zu7kJUia3rIuJTp93xA.

7. WebmateX (@SylvieWendlandt), "'Silly Cow' as Alf Garnet used to say….," Twitter, July 27, 2021, 1:01 p.m., https://twitter.com/SylvieWendlandt/status/1420066895512940549?s=20&t=Xb6Zu7kJUia3rIuJTp93xA.

8. Bethany George, "People Are Getting COVID Vaccine Tattoos to Celebrate Getting Their Shot," Yahoo! Finance, May 26, 2021, https://finance.yahoo.com/news/people-getting-covid-vaccine-tattoos-193026661.html; underbridged, Instagram, May 23, 2021, https://www.instag

ram.com/p/CPO743fD864/?utm_source=ig_embed&ig_rid=61ca8e18
-181a-4837-9407-d21e5b5dcbb2.

9. Ian Miller (@ianmSC), "Has anyone figured out yet why deaths . . . ,"
    Twitter, June 4, 2022, 3:23 p.m., https://twitter.com/ianmSC/status/15
    33167662364184576?s=20&t=y01xEqiydTkwRO1uIqHZdQ; Ian
    Miller, *Unmasked: The Global Failure of COVID Mask Mandates*
    (New York: Post Hill Press, 2022).

Chapter 10: Plexiglass Barriers in Stores and Businesses Save Lives! WRONG.

1. "2019 Performance Enabled Independent Grocer Success amid
    Pandemic," National Grocers Association, August 12, 2020, https://
    www.nationalgrocers.org/news/2019-performance-enabled-independe
    nt-grocer-success-amid-pandemic/.

2. Angela Eykelbosh, "A Rapid Review of the Use of Physical Barriers in
    Non-Clinical Settings and COVID-19 Transmission," National
    Collaborating Centre for Environmental Health, November 17, 2021,
    https://ncceh.ca/documents/evidence-review/rapid-review-use-physical
    -barriers-non-clinical-settings-and-covid-19; Carey Goldberg, "Plexiglass
    Is Everywhere, with No Proof It Keeps Covid at Bay," Bloomberg, June
    8, 2021, https://www.bloomberg.com/news/articles/2021-06-08/fortun
    es-spent-on-plastic-shields-with-no-proof-they-stop-covid; Tara Parker-
    Pope, "Those Anti-Covid Plastic Barriers Probably Don't Help and May
    Make Things Worse," *New York Times*, August 19, 2021, https://www
    .nytimes.com/2021/08/19/well/live/coronavirus-restaurants-classrooms
    -salons.html.

3. Neil Vigdor, "Fatal Accident with Metal Straw Highlights a Risk," *New
    York Times*, July 11, 2019, https://www.nytimes.com/2019/07/11/wor
    ld/europe/metal-straws-death.html.

4. "Tonnes of COVID-19 Health Care Waste Expose Urgent Need to
    Improve Waste Management Systems," World Health Organization,
    February 1, 2022, https://www.who.int/news/item/01-02-2022-tonnes

-of-covid-19-health-care-waste-expose-urgent-need-to-improve-waste
-management-systems; Julie Majdalani, "COVID Helped Increase
Medical Waste, Threatening People and Planet," Middle East Economy,
May 25, 2022, https://economymiddleeast.com/news/medical-waste/.

Chapter 11: Keeping People Inside and Locked Down Saves Lives! WRONG.

1. Trump White House Archived, "4/23/20: Members of the Coronavirus
    Task Force Hold a Press Briefing," YouTube, April 23, 2020, https://
    youtu.be/PsQnfpfIa_0?t=1187.
2. Denis Slattery, "'Shocking': 66% of New Coronavirus Patients in N.Y.
    Stayed Home: Cuomo," *New York Daily News*, May 6, 2020, https://
    www.nydailynews.com/coronavirus/ny-coronavirus-cuomo-coronavir
    us-stats-20200506-eyqui4b5lfdn7g6cqswkf6otly-story.html; CNBC
    Television, "New York Gov. Cuomo Holds a Briefing on the Coronavirus
    Outbreak—5/6/2020," YouTube, May 6, 2020, https://www.youtube
    .com/watch?v=8VZ_c-rbTHA.
3. T. Chad Baird (@TChadBaird), "What I see is a healthy middle age
    man…," Twitter, February 3, 2021, 3:56 p.m., https://twitter.com
    /TChadBaird/status/1357085606061375488.
4. Shruti Singh et al., "Prevalence of Low Level of Vitamin D among
    COVID-19 Patients and Associated Risk Factors in India—A Hospital-
    Based Study," *International Journal of General Medicine* 14 (June
    2021): 2523–31, https://www.ncbi.nlm.nih.gov/pmc/articles/PMC8214
    516/; "Vitamin D, Obesity and COVID-19," UC Health, January 31,
    2021, https://www.uchealth.com/en/media-room/covid-19/vitamin-d-o
    besity-and-covid-19; Guan Yu Lim, "Vitamin D Deficiency, Obesity and
    Diabetes Linked to Higher Rates of COVID-19 Infection and Mortality
    in Asia—Review," NutraIngredients-Asia, March 23, 2021, https://www
    .nutraingredients-asia.com/Article/2021/03/23/Vitamin-D-deficiency-ob
    esity-and-diabetes-linked-to-higher-rates-of-COVID-19-infection-and
    -mortality-in-Asia-Review; Dana K. Cassell, "New Study Found 80%

of COVID-19 Patients Were Vitamin D Deficient," Healthline, October 27, 2020, https://www.healthline.com/health-news/new-study-found-80 -percent-of-covid-19-patients-were-vitamin-d-deficient; Ray Marks, "Obesity, COVID-19 and Vitamin D: Is There an Association Worth Examining?," *Advances in Obesity, Weight Management & Control* 10, no. 3 (2020): 59–63, https://medcraveonline.com/AOWMC/obesity -covid-19-and-vitamin-d-is-there-an-association-worth-examining.html.

Chapter 12: Vax Mandates Save Lives! WRONG.

1. Aayushi Pratap, "Fauci: Covid-19 Vaccines Unlikely to Be Mandatory," *Forbes*, August 18, 2020, https://www.forbes.com/sites/aayushipratap /2020/08/18/fauci-covid-19-vaccines-unlikely-to-be-mandatory/?sh=37 a895195a01.

2. In August 2021 we tweeted out several points along these lines:
    Here's what's going to happen:
    Cases in Florida and most of the Sunbelt will subside.
    Cases will grow in the northeast.
    The FDA will give full approval to vaccines.
    Federal, state, school, and business vaccination mandates roll out with force.
    Late summer the "waning" will appear, and boosters will be needed! Justin Hart (@justin_hart), "Here's what's going to happen …," Twitter, August 5, 2021, 4:25 p.m., https://twitter.com/justin_hart/status/14233 94660165197824.

3. Justin Hart, "Pfizer Doc Revelations: Some Serious Concerns for Younger Cohorts," American Liberty News, March 8, 2022, https:// www.americanliberty.news/commentary/pfizer-doc-revelations-some -serious-concerns-for-younger-cohorts/jhart/2022/03/.

4. CDC (@CDCgov), "#DYK: VAERS data alone cannot show that an adverse…," Twitter, September 22, 2021, 1:15 p.m., https://twitter.com /CDCgov/status/1440726386226782213; Justin Hart (@justin_hart), "Oh look. Here's the CDC…," January 2, 2022, 2:32 p.m., https://tw

itter.com/justin_hart/status/1477724393300062208?s=20&t=qiD77Z
I7DRMJaZzrMsZIGQ.

5. Captured for our record here we have compiled a sample of adverse
    reactions among children:

    11 year old female—5 minutes post 1st dose said she couldn't hear,
    said she "couldn't feel her ears" Lost consciousness, came to after ~2–5
    minutes after—Had a seizure for 5 minutes Screamed for Mom to "Make
    it Stop"

    5 year old girl—IN—39 days post (unclear if 1st/2nd) dose Pfizer.—6
    days in hospital. Unclear if 1st/2nd—11/16/21. C19+ on 11/29/21 (symp
    onset 11/25/21). C19+ 13 days post [vaccine] MIS-C symptom onset
    12/25/21. Hospital for 6 days (MIS-C) confirmed case, onset 12/25/21.

    5 year old girl—AZ—4 days post unknown dose Pfizer—5 days in
    hospital C19+ October Vax 4 weeks later MIS-C "Pt had acute acute
    COVID19 in October 2021. Got her first COVID19 vaccine on 11/12/21.
    Started having fever on 11/16/21 & was admitted on 11/21/21 w/MIS-C
    with Cardiac involvement"

    10 year old girl—AR—41 days post 1st dose Pfizer—2 days in the
    hospital Ketoacidosis Type 1 Diabetes Mellitus Pollakiuria "Child began
    deep thirst and urination on January 10. Rushed to hospital on January
    11th and subsequently diagnosed with Type 1 Diabetes."

    7 year old boy—TN—43 days post unknown dose Pfizer—Unknown
    days in hospital MIS-C Lymphadenitis Conjunctivitis Strawberry Tongue
    "On 02/15/2022 patient presented to hospital with concerns for MIS-C;
    developed fevers, tmax of 105F, also complained of myalgia, and
    abdominal pain."

    5 year old boy—PR—13 days post 2nd dose Pfizer—Lymphadenitis
    Movement Disorder Tic "Tic disorder Repetitive neck movements
    developed after 12 days of vaccine administration He had a cervical
    lymphadenitis developed on left anterior neck after vaccine as described
    by mother"

5 year old boy—IN—19 days post 1st dose Pfizer—2 days in hospital (would be labeled "unvaccinated" per CDC definitions) MIS-C C19+ (19 days post vax) "Multisystem Inflammatory Syndrome confirmed case, onset 12/13/21" "12/20/2021 SARS-CoV-2 IgG Ab positive"

8 year old boy—NY—33 days post unknown dose Pfizer—3 days in hospital (unclear which way he would be labeled) Immune Thrombocytopenia 1/10/22—CBC showed platelet count of less than 1. 1/11/22—IVIG administered CBC showed platelet count of 5 1/12/22—CBC showed platelet count of < 1

5 year old girl—NY—1 day post unknown dose Pfizer—(10 mcgm w/Tris) 3 days in hospital Seizure Foaming at the Mouth Pineal Gland Cyst "Seizure event possibly longer than 15 minutes. Mother found her slumped over in bed w/foaming at the mouth. +postictal state. She did have a fever"

16 year old male—NY—9 days post 1st dose Pfizer—2 days in hospital Would be labeled "unvaxxed" per CDC definitions Tonic-Clonic Seizure Postictal State Event on 9/10/21 Reported 2/3/22

8 year old boy—19 days post 1st dose Pfizer—(10 mcgm w/Tris) Epilepsy Intractable Seizures EEG Severely Abnormal "intractable seizures was loaded with anti seizure meds in ER and admitted to the hospital to further get seizures under control"

5 year old girl—5 days post 1st dose Pfizer—(10 mcgm w/Tris) Seizure lasting 2 minutes 2nd Seizure 6 days later EKG Abnormal "Seizure on 11/23/21 and seizure on 11/29/21, each lasting approximately 2 minutes. EEG found abnormal . Started medication for seizures on 12/1/21"

7 year old boy—1 day post 2nd dose Pfizer—(10 mcgm w/Tris) Seizure "he had a seizure (right hand posturing, body turned to left, emesis & turned blue, he gasped) àthis lasted 4–5 minutes. Emergency was called & in ambulance, he had a 2nd witnessed tonic clonic seizure w/eyes deviated"

6 year old girl—7 days post 1st dose Pfizer—(10 mcgm w/Tris) 2 days in hospital Seizure Loss of Consciousness "All test results have come back

normal at this time and care providers cannot identify another causal factor for the seizure." Encourage a read of all of the verbiage.

5 year old boy—3 days post Unknownnown Dose Pfizer—(10 mcgm w/Tris) Seizure "The fever increased to 101, a dose of Tylenol was given, and about 10 minutes later he had a seizure lasting ~3.5 minutes at 3:45pm. An ambulance was called and he was taken to the hospital. Temp in ER was 102."

5 year old boy—10 hours post 2nd dose Pfizer—(10 mcgm w/Tris) Seizure Gaze Palsy "No patient or family history of seizure conditions. Child was unresponsive for 1–3 minutes with eyes open and fixed, mouth open, arms and legs extended and muscles rigid and twitching."

12 year old male—6 days post 1st dose Pfizer—(30 mcgm PBS) Seizure "He had just begun to brush his teeth when he collapsed and had a seizure. He has no medical reason to have seizures & had never had one until 6 days after getting the vaccine."

6 year old girl—7 days post 1st dose Pfizer—(10 mcgm w/Tris) Seizure "Child had seizure (lost consciousness and stopped breathing) 1 week after 1st dose of Pfizer COVID-19 vaccine. Child was transported via ambulance to hospital where she was admitted & will be spending the night."...

7 year old female—8 days post 1st dose Pfizer—(10 mcgms w/Tris) Multiple Seizures 2 days in hospital No significant prior medical history

13 year old female—5–6 days post 2nd dose Pfizer—38 days in the hospital Encephalitis Prior, she had been previously healthy and developmentally normal...In addition to seizure, she has become nonverbal, unable to eat, and does not follow commands.

21 year old female—Right after 1st dose Pfizer—Peri Paralysis Seizure LP 7 days in hospital "I was pretty much paralyzed for hands and legs. I was brought to hospital and they treated me there for about a week and I had muscle weakness I gained feeling back in my hands but not in my feet"

18 year old female—10 days post 2nd Pfizer—Hospital 3 days "Pt w/ seizures & encephalitis 10 days after 2nd C19 vaccine No source of encephalitis was found, although workup continues Pt is recovering but still has extreme fatigue & decreased functioning including decreased mental stamina

14 year old female—7 days post 1st dose Pfizer—Grand Mal Seizure "a generalized tonic-clonic seizure—is caused by abnormal electrical activity throughout the brain." Hospitalized for unknownnown days

12 year old female—NJ—5 days post 2nd dose Pfizer—Would be labeled as "unvaccinated" in the hospital 11 days in the hospital MIS-C Pt was admit 11/30/21 because of concern for septic shock. Pt is a 12 year old female prev healthy, presenting w/a 6 day history of abdom pain & febrile illness

12 year old female—TX—13 days post—2nd dose Pfizer hospital 3 times, 7–10 days each time Acute Pyelonephritis Kidney Infection UTIs Muscle Spasms Renal Disorder Encourage a read of all of the verbiage.

12 year old male—IA—12 days post 3rd dose Pfizer—Immune Thrombocytopenia "Patient was diagnosed with Immune thrombocytopenia by local hospital" "CBC w/dif, Reticulocytes done on 2/3/22 at local Clinic. PT, PTT, INR, CRP, Ferritin, UA, repeat CBC done 2/3/22 @ local hospital"

12 year old female—CA—1 day post 2nd dose—Pfizer Glossitis (Swollen Tongue) "Sore arm, Fever (103 degree), bumps on tongue (painful), tongue and cheek swelling, roof of mouth swelling, sore gum. Diagnosed with Glossitis. Prescribed steroids, pain medication, and Benedryl."

17 year old female—MN—1 month post 2nd dose Pfizer—Immune Thrombocytopenia "(07/08/21) my platelets were at 53,000 I have had 39 blood tests to date to monitor my platelets. They have fluctuated up and down due to ongoing steroid treatment (12/21/21) my platelets were @ 66,000"

12 year old female—GA—10 days post 2nd dose Pfizer—8 months post vax still ongoing papilledema "Pt was dx w/papilledema of both eyes. Prev eye exams & dilated exam do not reflect papilledema. Multiple specialists cannot uncover the cause...8 months later it has not resolved."

13 year old female—7 day—post 1st dose Pfizer Brain Natriuretic Peptide Increased PICU for potential Myocarditis Chest Pain "Came to the ER on 12/24 with intermittent chest pain that started 12/23 after she played soccer."

15 year old female—177 post 2nd dose of Pfizer—Bilateral Pulmonary Emboli Autopsy Pending. "Patient passed away on 12/11/21 at 12:11pm from bilateral pulmonary emboli (air bubbles not DVT). Final autopsy results pending toxicology results."

12 year old female—7 days post 2nd dose Pfizer—Went to ER Immune Thrombocytopenia Haemoglobin Decrease "Placed under hemotology care. Child was diagnosed w/iron deficiency and ITP (Immuno thrombocytopenia) We were sent to Institute. Child platelets kept dropping"

12 year old female—1 day post 2nd dose Pfizer—5 days in the hospital Autoimmune Haemolytic Anemia Jaundice Platelet Count Decreased "At the er they diagnosed her w/autoimmune hemolytic anemia, which explained the jaundice She was admitted & put on steroids Her hemoglobin got as low as 5"

12 year old female—2 days post dose. Acute Promyelocytic Leukemia (usually occurs in those ~40) 5 days in hospital Leukocytosis Thrombocytopenia Leg pain and bruising. Fever right after vax, initially thought to be appendicitis.

BOOSTER—DEATH—17 year old male—Foreign—8 days post 3rd dose Pfizer—onset of symptoms hospitalized 15 days post 3rd dose Pfizer—DEAD Agranulocytosis Sepsis Multiple Organ Dysfunction Syndrome

16 year old male—TX—4 days post 1st dose Pfizer—20 days in hospital (over 4 different periods) Chronic Inflammatory Demyelinating

Polyneuropathy Immunoglobulin Therapy "Chronic Inflammatory Demyelinating Polyneuropathy Patient hospitalized several times for IVIG treatments"

16 year old male—NY—9 days post 1st dose Pfizer—2 days in hospital Would be labeled "unvaxxed" per CDC definitions Tonic-Clonic Seizure Postictal State Event on 9/10/21 Reported 2/3/22

And that's the just the tip of the iceberg. This list is from Justin Hart, "Screamed for Mom to 'Make it Stop,'" Rational Ground (Substack), March 8, 2022, https://covidreason.substack.com/p/screamed-for-mom-to-make-it-stop?s=w; adverse reactions compiled from OpenVAERS, https://openvaers.com/.

6.   Greg Hunter's USAWatchdog.com, "CV19 Vax Deadliest Fraud in History—Edward Dowd," Rumble, June 7, 2022, https://rumble.com/v17omi3-cv19-vax-deadliest-fraud-in-history-edward-dowd.html. This is daunting and depressing stuff, of course. At times, this would prove too much for many of our colleagues. They would sign off for months to regain composure. Constantly kicking against a seemingly immovable object can be exhausting. We found that humor was one of the key tactics to reaching the minds of folks who were slowly being "red-pilled" into the reality of what we were experiencing.

To convey the ridiculousness of the growing number of boosters needed to demonstrate full vaccination, we composed a fake vaccine "loyalty" booster card—like a sandwich shop. When you fill up all ten boosters you get a free Fauci plush doll (those *do* actually exist by the way).

On another occasion we made light of the FDA's recommendation that one could sign up for a host of different vaccines to try and boost immunity. In October 2021 the FDA suggested that people could couple vaccine doses together to achieve even *better* efficacy. To help our enthusiastic friends along, we put together a quick cocktail menu named after four big members of Team Apocalypse. Dr. Tony Fauci, Andy Slavitt,

CDC director Rochelle Walensky, and Pfizer board member Scott Gottlieb.

FAUCI FRESCA: 2 shots of deep freezer-borne Moderna plus 1 shot of Pfizer's best (hold the J&J)

SLAVITT SIPPER: The works! J&J double with a 2 oz. Moderna on the rocks topped with a squeeze of Pfizer

WALENSKY WINE COOLER: Drink with a twist! Promising a maskless, infection-less experience then a rug-pull to reveal a leaky vaccine.

GOTTLIEB GOBBLER: Public/private blend. Sweet aroma of cashing in on connections. Pure Pfizer straight up plus 10 boosters.

Levity, satire, and parody were just some of the many tactics we used to convey topics that might otherwise be boring or go unnoticed. It also helped us keep our sanity in the face of serious harms to adults and children brushed under the carpet.

7. Pajamas It Is (@HeckofaLiberal), "THREAD: For those still claiming…," (thread) Twitter, July 26, 2020, 8:45 p.m., https://twitter.com/Hec kofaLiberal/status/1287549725567197184?s=20&t=qiD77ZI7DRMJ aZzrMsZIGQ.

8. Julia Belluz, "Long Covid Isn't as Unique as We Thought," *Vox*, April 7, 2021, https://www.vox.com/22298751/long-term-side-effects-covid -19-hauler-symptoms.

Chapter 13: Natural Immunity Is Not an Alternative to Vaccination! WRONG.

1. "Washington Journal: Influenza Vaccine," C-SPAN, October 11, 2004, https://www.c-span.org/video/?183885-2/influenza-vaccine.

2. Reid Wilson, "Health Experts Say 'Herd Immunity' Strategy Would Kill Thousands," *The Hill*, October 16, 2021, https://thehill.com/policy/hea lthcare/521259-health-experts-say-herd-immunity-strategy-would-kill -thousands/.

3.   "Why COVID-19 Vaccines Should Not Be Required for All Americans,"
     U.S. News & World Report, August 5, 2021, https://www.usnews.com/
     news/national-news/why-covid-19-vaccines-should-not-be-requir
     ed-for-all-americans.

4.   Here are a sample of quotes from various studies confirming natural
     immunity as a viable, even superior, protection approach to
     COVID-19.

     "Natural immunity confers longer-lasting and stronger protection
     against infection, symptomatic disease and hospitalization caused by the
     Delta variant of SCoV2, compared to vaccine-induced immunity."
     (medRxiv)

     "Israelis who had an infection were more protected against the Delta
     coronavirus variant than those who had an already highly effective
     COVID-19 vaccine." (*Science*)

     The NIH posts this: "The immune systems of more than 95% of
     people who recovered from COVID19 had durable memories of the virus
     up to eight months after infection." (*Science*)

     Out of Ireland: "Reinfection was an uncommon event (absolute rate
     0%–1.1%), with no study reporting an increase in the risk of reinfection
     over time." (*JAMA* Network)

     Denmark: "The spike protein was identified as the dominant target
     for both neutralizing antibodies and T-cell responses. Overall, the
     majority of patients had robust adaptive immune responses, regardless of
     their disease severity." (*The Lancet*)

     From the UK: "T-cell responses were present in all [non-hospitalized]
     individuals at six months after SARS-CoV-2 infection." (UK-CIC)

     From Emory University: "Our findings show that most C19 patients
     induce a wide-ranging immune defense against SARS-CoV-2 infection,
     encompassing antibodies and memory B cells recognizing both the RBD
     and other regions of the spike..." (Cell.com)

Washington University and Nature: "Our results indicate that mild infection with SCoV2 induces robust antigen-specific, long-lived humoral immune memory in humans." (*Nature*)

This list is from Justin Hart, "Your Natural Immunity Cheat Sheet," Rational Ground (Substack), October 10, 2021, https://covidreason.sub stack.com/p/your-natural-immunity-cheat-sheet.

Chapter 14: Children Are Resilient and Will Bounce Back! WRONG.

1. "New CDC Data Nationally Representative Survey of High School Students during the Pandemic Can Inform Effective Programs," Centers for Disease Control and Prevention, March 31, 2022, https://www.cdc .gov/media/releases/2022/p0331-youth-mental-health-covid-19.html; "Emergency Department Visits for Suspected Suicide Attempts among Persons Aged 12–25 Years before and during the COVID-19 Pandemic— United States, January 2019–May 2021," Centers for Disease Control and Prevention, June 18, 2021, https://www.cdc.gov/mmwr/volumes/70 /wr/mm7024e1.htm.

2. David Zweig, "New Research Suggests Number of Kids Hospitalized for COVID Is Overcounted," Intelligencer, May 19, 2021, https://nym ag.com/intelligencer/2021/05/study-number-of-kids-hospitalized-for-co vid-is-overcounted.html.

3. Mark Kelly, "Palm Beach Therapist Sees Increase in Children's Speech Delays during COVID-19," ABC WPBF 25 News, November 9, 2021, https://www.wpbf.com/article/palm-beach-covid-therapist-speech- delays/38189805#.

Chapter 15: Children Are Walking Vectors of Disease! WRONG.

1. Preferred Protective Equipment, "Back To School Safely—Student Ultralite Total Comfort Face Shield | Preferred Protective Equipment,"

YouTube, August 6, 2020, https://www.youtube.com/watch?v=V-yk2k
bkiNk&list=TLGGX90dqTEgfr4yNzA2MjAyMg&t=29s.

2. Justin Hart (@justin_hart), "We've lost our ever-lovin' minds!…,"
Twitter, September 21, 2020, 11:23 p.m., https://twitter.com/justin_ha
rt/status/1308245550878269444?s=20&t=oKoceMkw8eY7Ljienn
QZrw.

3. Faye Brown, "Students with Corona Told 'Stay in Rooms a Minute
Longer' If There's a Fire in Halls," *Metro*, October 15, 2020, https://me
tro.co.uk/2020/10/15/students-with-corona-told-stay-in-rooms-a-minu
te-longer-if-theres-a-fire-in-halls-13425345/?ito=article.amp.share.top
.twitter.

4. Justin Hart (@justin_hart), "We've lost our everlovin' minds.…," Twitter,
October 11, 2020, 12:24 p.m., https://twitter.com/justin_hart/status/1
315327499039956994?s=20.

5. Dawn Reiss, "Chicago Teachers Balk at Reopening Plan, Face Pay Loss
If They Don't Return," *Washington Post*, January 9, 2021, https://www
.washingtonpost.com/local/education/chicago-public-schools-reopen-pl
an/2021/01/09/e2e7f5a6-5286-11eb-83e3-322644d82356_story.html.

6. One of the Rational Ground followers on Twitter, @RayPrisament,
devised an excellent thread cataloguing the impact on kids of wearing
masks. The thread include reports such as the following:

New York Times: "Masks have encouraged anonymity and discouraged
dialogue."

"'People don't know how to communicate anymore,' said Jazlyn
Korpics, 18, a senior at Liberty. 'Everybody's a robot now—their minds
are warped.'"

WSJ: "Facial expressions are integral to human connection,
particularly for young children…. Covering a child's face mutes these
nonverbal forms of communication and can result in robotic and
emotionless interactions."

Professor Emily Oster: "The concerns here stem from the observation
that the bottom half of the face is important for reading emotions,

learning to speak, and learning to read. The theory behind this is compelling."

"Masks are not a friendship bracelet"

New York Times: "Masks can impede communication"

Boston Globe: "[Mask-free] students reported 'happier hallways,' 'contagious smiling,' and better class discussions. With fewer masks, English language learners and students learning foreign languages reported better communication."

Tablet: "Fifty-nine percent of U.K. teachers in April 2021 stated that asking pupils to wear masks made understanding them a 'lot more difficult.' We know that when someone conceals their lips it's harder to comprehend what they're saying."

RayPrisament (@RayPrisament), "Oh no, you didn't just say masks on kids . . . ," (thread) Twitter, January 21, 2022, 6:14 p.m., https://twitter.com/RayPrisament/status/1484665648223510529.

Chapter 16: School Closures Are a Necessary Step to Save Lives! WRONG.

1. AJ Kay (@AJKayWriter), "My autistic daughter's private school . . . ," Twitter, November 24, 2020, 10:06 a.m., https://twitter.com/AJKayWriter/status/1331252890120327170?s=20&t=qiD77ZI7DRMJaZzrMsZIGQ.

2. Ms. Katie (@CTUSpecialEd), "Our PreK team was told to report . . . ," Twitter, January 4, 2021, 9:54 a.m., https://twitter.com/CTUSpecialEd/status/1346107776678961154?s=20&t=qiD77ZI7DRMJaZzrMsZIGQ.

3. Suzanne Downing, "Class Warfare: Students in Anchorage Will Be Forced to Kneel for Hours, No Recess," Must Read Alaska, January 19, 2021, https://mustreadalaska.com/class-warfare-students-in-anchorage-will-be-forced-to-kneel-for-hours-no-recess/.

4. Matt Malkus (@malkusm), "This is the inside of an MNPS 'virtual learning center,' where students . . . ," Twitter, January 21, 2021, 10:30

a.m., https://twitter.com/malkusm/status/1352277465947926531?s=2 0&t=Zv6d6A4mqkuMJeVOdCELgQ.

5. Mom On A Mission #singleissuevoter (@MomOnAMission30), "I find this picture so sad. . . . ," Twitter, February 17, 2021, 8:58 p.m., https:// twitter.com/MomOnAMission30/status/1362219900140421125?s=20.

6. Laura "Summer of Joy" Lynn (@LauraLynn209), "From band instructor in Minooka IL D201. . . . ," Twitter, August 4, 2021, 10:13 p.m., https:// twitter.com/LauraLynn209/status/1423104801269747712?s=20&t=e q8ohUr2_CoIq4r9IQJLeA.

7. Laura "Summer of Joy" Lynn (@LauraLynn209), "From Illinois School District 207...," Twitter, March 4, 2021, 6:03 p.m., https://twitter.com /LauraLynn209/status/1367611758660235265?s=20&t=eq8ohUr2_Co Iq4r9IQJLeA.

8. Moms for Liberty (@Moms4Liberty), "Apparently breathing oxygen is now considered a reward...," Twitter, May 7, 2021, 7:14 a.m., https:// twitter.com/Moms4Liberty/status/1390626144504930304?s=20.

9. Jon Brown, "Colorado Bus Driver Admits to Slapping 10-Year-Old Girl in Face over Mask," Daily Wire+, May 20, 2021, https://www.dailywire. com/news/colorado-bus-driver-admits-to-slapping-10-year-old-girl-in-face-over-mask; Ashley Franco, "CAUGHT ON CAMERA: Colorado School Bus Driver Accused of Slapping a Child for Not Wearing a Mask Properly," KKTV11 News, May 17, 2021, https://www.kktv .com/2021/05/18/colorado-bus-driver-facing-charges-for-allegedly-slap ping-kid-over-mask/.

10. Antigone Michaelides (oneantigone), "My son, Leo, now age 10, at the Metropolitan Opera...," Twitter, July 30, 2021, 11:28 a.m., https://tw itter.com/oneantigone/status/1421130500870221831?s=20&t=Nl3sNl 2CbmsP8VZfLvFL-A.

Chapter 17: Lockdowns Keep Kids Alive! WRONG.

1. Robert Preidt, "Child Drownings in U.S. Pools, Spas Are on the Rise," HealthDay, June 10, 2021, https://consumer.healthday.com/child-drow nings-in-u-s-pools-spas-are-on-the-rise-2653294591.html.

2. Sebastian Mader and Tobias Rüttenauer, "The Effects of Non-Pharmaceutical Interventions on COVID-19 Mortality: A Generalized Synthetic Control Approach across 169 Countries," *Frontiers in Public Health* 10 (April 4, 2022), https://www.frontiersin.org/articles/10.3389 /fpubh.2022.820642/full.

3. "Learning Losses from COVID-19 Could Cost This Generation of Students Close to $17 Trillion in Lifetime Earnings," UNICEF, December 6, 2021, https://www.unicef.org/press-releases/learning-losses-covid-19 -could-cost-generation-students-close-17-trillion-lifetime; "The State of the Global Education Crisis: A Path to Recovery," World Bank, December 3, 2021, https://www.worldbank.org/en/topic/education/pub lication/the-state-of-the-global-education-crisis-a-path-to-recovery; Helen Raleigh, "Shocking Data Shows School Closures Caused Severe Learning Loss for Children around the Globe," The Federalist, March 24, 2022, https://thefederalist.com/2022/03/24/shocking-data-shows-sc hool-closures-caused-severe-learning-loss-for-children-around-the-gl obe/.

4. Raleigh, "Shocking Data Shows."

5. Dan Goldhaber, Thomas J. Kane, and Andrew McEachin, "Analysis: Pandemic Learning Loss Could Cost U.S. Students $2 Trillion in Lifetime Earnings. What States & Schools Can Do to Avert This Crisis," The 74, December 13, 2021, https://www.the74million.org/article/analysis-pandemic-learning-loss-could-cost-u-s-students-2-trillion-in-lifetime-earnings-what-states-schools-can-do-to-avert-this-crisis/; Karyn Lewis and Megan Kuhfeld, "Learning during COVID-19: An Update on Student Achievement and Growth at the Start of the 2021–22 School Year," Center for School and Student Progress, December 2021, https://www.nwea.org/content/uploads/2021/12/Learning-during-CO

VID19-An-update-on-student-achievement-and-growth-at-the-start-of
-the-2021-2022-school-year-Research-Brief.pdf.

Chapter 18: Teachers and Schools Were Hardest Hit by the Lockdowns! WRONG.

1. "Burbio ESSER III Spending Tracker," Burbio, 2022, https://info.burb
    io.com/esser-iii-spending/.

2. Our friends at Burbio, an education-focused school calendaring software
    company, turned their eye towards tracking Covid data. Here's just a
    sample of the type of outlays they've documented. The school district is
    listed, and the amount allocated is in the parentheses which follow:

    Jonesboro School District, AR ($20.6MM) will be spending $4.8MM
    on "Additional Pay: COVID-19 related expenditures related to preventing
    disruptions and closures. Recruitment and retention of a diverse and
    qualified educator workforce."

    Alum Rock Union Elementary School District, CA ($22.5MM) will
    be spending just under $18MM on "Staff recruitment, support and
    retention/Costs related to providing direct support to students." Of the
    total, $8.1MM is targeted to "Retention of staff to ensure continuity of
    learning—Administrators" and $9.8 MM to "Retention of staff to ensure
    continuity of learning-Support Staff." Fontana Unified School District,
    CA ($96MM) is spending $24.1MM: "Additional monetary one-time
    compensation will be provided to all staff for the 2021–22 for school-
    related duties attributable to transitioning to full-person instruction with
    virtual instructional options as well as implementing COVID-19 safety
    practices and procedures."

    Portland Public Schools, ME ($17.9MM) will spend $6.3MM on
    "Salary, benefits, stipends and related pay for educational staff
    ($6,000,000), as well as vaccination bonuses for vaccinated staff to ensure
    the safety of our staff and students ($275,000)" this year.

Socorro Consolidated Schools, NM ($6.7MM) will be spending just over $3MM to "Pay retention/recruitment/hazard payment to all staff who are employed now and attract new staff for open positions."

Checotah Public Schools, OK ($3.1MM) "plans to use ESSER III funds to provide return to work stipends, hazard duty stipends, and training stipends for 2022FY, 2023FY, and 2024FY. We project that the stipends will cost a total of $1,116,000.00 for all three fiscal years. These stipends will help retain employees in the current climate that they are asked to work in. It will also allow the school to train the employees in COVID prevention measures." Meanwhile Tulsa Public Schools, OK ($130.8MM) is planning on $10MM for "Recruitment and retention incentives to ensure continuity of service to students and staff and fill hard-to-staff roles and schools."

Bend-La Pine Schools, OR ($18.8MM) is spending $2.4MM to "provide distinguished service stipends for all BLS staff."

Roma ISD, TX ($33.7MM) will be spending $4MM per year over the next three years for "Staff Retention Stipends."

Greenbriar County Schools, WV ($13MM) will be using $9.6MM to retain staff between now and 2024: "To combat student achievement gaps, students will benefit from smaller class sizes due to achievement and social/emotional regulation gaps due to COVID 19. We do not yet know how our enrollment will pan out with some families choosing homeschooling when remote learning is no longer an option. Virtual school will still be an option." Hardy County Schools, WV ($4.9MM) is spending $422,000 on retaining staff.

Winner School District, SD ($3.3MM) is "looking at" paying $750 incentive bonuses at the end of each semester, for a total cost of $150,000.

Mount Ida School District, AR ($1.5MM) is spending $326,802 on "additional demands—compensation" in addition to $117,000 on "COVID leave."

Washakie County School District # 1, WY ($4MM) has set aside $775,600 for "workforce stabilization."

This list is from "K-12 School Reopening Trends," Burbio, April 18, 2022, https://info.burbio.com/school-tracker-update-4-18-22/.

3.   Examples include:

Fort Worth ISD, TX ($262MM) will be adding 107 full time family engagement specialists at all elementary and middle schools whose responsibilities will include "attendance monitoring, customer service (welcoming school environment), volunteer management, social media management, social emotional learning support and crisis intervention, parent advocacy, site based decision making and understanding assessment data."

Guilford County School, NC ($198MM), which reports an enrollment drop from 73,321 in 2017/18 to 70,227 in 2020/21, gives details on their plans: "Employ public relations firm to assist with PK marketing to increase enrollment—Student and family community liaisons and college transition counselors to support students who need support with attendance/engagement—Weekly student level Canvas reporting tools and dashboards for schools to identify students who need support... Counselor and social worker training sessions for utilizing data sources... Weekly logs to track services for Students with Disabilities and English Learners—Student support committees.... Attendance campaign through partnership with Attendance Works..."

Allentown School District, PA ($88MM) outlines multiple approaches: "Hire Learning Loss Attendance Support Specialists to work closely with attendance teams and assist schools with attendance intervention/ strategies to improve attendance using school specific attendance data analysis and evidence-based strategy planning to.... encourage re-engagement and reduce truancy and learning loss;" "Hire Community Aides to visit and communicate with families, encourage engagement, align families with the necessary staff/support and verify residency;" "Offer the Continuum of services/supports for students and families experiencing homelessness;" and "Implement Attendance Outreach

Initiatives, such as our Attendance Outreach Campaign, to re-engage students who are chronically absent."

District of Columbia Public Schools, Washington, DC ($193MM) outlines a wide variety of engagement-related policies in their Continuous Education plan for this current year. Among several initiatives outlined, we noted the following: 1) A "Confidence Campaign" featuring school level outreach and engagement, a digital content and storytelling strategy to reach stakeholders, and health and education delivered both virtually and in-person to address questions and concerns. 2) Ongoing two-way communication objectives with parents with regard to their students' progress activated at the school level 3) Outreach to students who were disengaged from virtual learning as well as chronically absent "from school-based attendance counselors, teachers, school leaders, DCPS Central Services, and from external partners like Child and Family Services Agency (CFSA) when necessary. DCPS updated our unexcused absence notification process to include a wellness call after three days of unexcused absences."

Marlboro County School District, SC ($19.9MM) will implement the following: 1) Care closets will be placed in each school to provide students unable to meet, or have limited access to, such basic needs as toiletries and clothing. 2) Implementation of an evening program offering classes for high school graduation and/or GED, targeted to students who have entered the workforce. 3) Fifteen "Living Learning Resource Centers" will be established around the County located in churches, community centers, and housing authorities. "The project will include the purchase of computers, furniture, carpet and paint."

Granite School District, UT ($97.5MM) will spend $500,000 on "Student attendance supports and initiatives to improve daily attendance" with a goal to "return (to) or exceed" pre-Covid 19 attendance levels. In addition, in an area of support we see in many plans, the district will spend $1MM on "Improved parent engagement initiatives so parents know how they can effectively support their student(s);" metrics to be measured for success of this initiative include the "number of parents monitoring grades, attending school events, volunteering, etc." and the percent of parents setting up an account in the parent portal.

Hamilton County Schools, TN ($91MM) will allocate "Funds for Literacy Community Events to educate families and communities on Foundational Literacy Skills and to provide at-home literacy resources. Truancy Specialists will work with students, families, and the school to ensure students are at school and not truant. Mobile classrooms, Family Resource Specialist and advanced messaging services" will also be deployed.

This list is from Justin Hart, "Public School Enrollment: Abandoning the Cities," Rational Ground (Substack), April 11, 2022, https://covidreason.substack.com/p/public-school-enrollment-abandoning.

Covid funds for transportation are also interesting to review:

Worcester Public Schools, MA ($78.2MM), which voted to take its bus service in-house, is spending $18.5MM on school buses.

Minneapolis Public Schools, MN ($159.5MM) will be spending $2.4MM on bus driver recruitment and retention.

Lincoln County Schools, WV ($12MM) is spending $190,000 on a refrigerated food truck to bring food to students and families, plus $300,000 for wi-fi on buses. Similarly Truth or Consequences Municipal Schools, NM ($5.4MM) will spend $125,000 on a "mid-sized bus to help deliver meals to our remote students so we do not have to disrupt the regular bus schedule."

Wappingers Central School District, NY ($8.6MM) will spend $100,000 on additional bus driver hours, and have allocated $1MM for transportation for students for summer school and afterschool programs.

Crown Point Community School Corporation, IN ($3.9MM) will be spending over $200,000 in bus drivers' salary and benefits and bus fuel and maintenance in programs to address learning loss.

Frederick County Public Schools, MD ($37.9MM) will be using buses as Mobile Learning Labs. "These learning labs will visit a neighborhood twice a week, for one hour each visit, for an eight week session. Two sessions will occur—the first in fall 2021 and the second in spring 2022. Three teachers will participate in each learning lab session; materials for the session will be brought from their school..."

Riverbank Unified School District, CA ($6.3MM) is spending $40,000 on Transportation Recording Systems for "Cameras in buses to provide video information related to student interaction, connection and contact tracing."

Windham Public Schools, CT ($13.7MM) is spending $100,000 to purchase a Parent Transportation Van, with additional expenses for gas and staffing.

Hastings Public Schools, NE ($6.8MM) will be spending $775,000 on "buses and suburbans" this year and next, while Pryor Public Schools, OK ($4.4MM) will be spending $1.1MM on 6 buses and 6 suburbans. Dallas County Schools, AL ($21.9MM) will be spending $3MM on 30 72-passenger buses "to reduce the amount of students riding and to mitigate COVID 19 infection when transporting students."

Westmoreland County Public Schools, VA ($4.5MM) is spending $700,000 to purchase six air-conditioned buses to replace six non-air-conditioned buses, as well as $82,900 for bus cameras to assist in contact tracing.

Byers School District, CO ($2.7MM) will spend $226,000 to "Add vehicles for smaller travel" and spend $16,000 on bus wi-fi.

This is list is from "K-12 School Reopening Trends," Burbio, April 4, 2022, https://info.burbio.com/school-tracker-update-4-04-22/.

4. Examples include:

South Jefferson Central School District, NY ($5.6MM) will be spending just over $650,000 on over 5,000 pieces of classroom furniture across elementary, middle and high schools.

Lemoor Union Elementary CA ($6.5MM) will be spending $1MM on Outdoor Shade Structures to "provide outdoor spaces on each campus to spread students out in a safe manner and reduce or prevent the spread of COVID-19. In addition to grade level classrooms, PE, music, and afterschool programs will utilize these spaces to ensure safe distancing as well."

Amphitheater Public Schools, AZ ($29MM) will spend $800,000 to create an Internship Center at the high school, in addition to furniture purchases.

Hernando School District, FL ($43.6MM) will be spending $350,000 on air purification systems for school buses.

Huron School District, SD ($6.3MM) will be spending $750,000 on the addition of four outdoor tennis courts.

Omaha Public School, NE ($194MM) will be spending $43MM on roof replacements and $5MM on hydration stations.

Bloomfield Public Schools, CT ($3.5MM) will spending on two-way radios for school security and district leadership, outdoor seating for meal times for Special Education, and lunch tables for the high school to increase distancing during rush periods.

Laredo, TX ($123MM) is spending $11.6MM on fire and security alarm systems, $225,000 for water fountain retrofits for bottle fillers, $280,000 for electronic marquees, $43,000 for digital food temperature monitoring, $756,000 on security cameras, $2.4MM on school buses, and $160,000 for 8 sets of washers and dryers.

Kanawha County, WV ($82MM) is spending over $5MM on outdoor classroom materials, outdoor classroom improvements, window replacements for better ventilation, and improvements to bathrooms and flooring.

MSAD 53, Pittsfield, ME ($2.4MM) is spending on a family bathroom, outdoor bleachers, and improved cooling systems at the middle school, plus playground and bathroom upgrades.

Danville Public Schools, VA ($29.7MM) is spending $8.9MM to renovate an existing school building to reduce overcrowding and free up space for in-person learning across the district.

Albuquerque Public Schools, NM ($230MM) will be spending $4.9MM on water repiping and $6.8MM on window replacement.

This list is from "K-12 Reopening Trends," Burbio, March 21, 2022, https://info.burbio.com/school-tracker-update-3-21-22/.

5. Caroline Beetz Fenske, "Measuring Learning Loss from School Closures during the Pandemic and Beyond," Federal Reserve Bank of Chicago, August 19, 2021, https://www.chicagofed.org/publications/blogs/chicago-fed-insights/2021/measuring-learning-loss.

Chapter 19: School Reopenings Have Been Gradual but Effective! WRONG.

1. Reema Amin and Christina Veiga, "NYC's Homeschooling Option: Any Family Can Choose Full-Time Remote Learning This Fall," The City, July 2, 2020, https://www.thecity.nyc/2020/7/2/21312118/nyc-homeschooling-remote-learning-choice-fall.

2. Taryn Luna and Phil Willon, "Restaurant Dining Rooms, Wineries, Card Rooms to Close for at Least Three Weeks in 19 California Counties," *Los Angeles Times*, July 1, 2020, https://www.latimes.com/california/story/2020-07-01/newsom-imposes-new-rollbacks-of-californias-coronavirus-reopening.

3. Zachary Evans, "CDC Urges Schools to Reopen 'as Soon as Possible,' Says COVID Risk Can Be Mitigated," Yahoo! Sports, February 12, 2021, https://sports.yahoo.com/cdc-urges-schools-reopen-soon-195508598.html.

4. Jeffrey A. Tucker, "When Will the Madness End?," American Institute of Economic Research, July 10, 2020, https://www.aier.org/article/when-will-the-madness-end/.

Chapter 20: Your Behavior Can Stop the Virus! WRONG.

1. "Joe Rogan Joins the Anti-Fauci Revolution," Clay & Buck, August 18, 2021, https://www.clayandbuck.com/joe-rogan-joins-the-anti-fauci-rev olution/.

2. NewsTime, "Blackrock CEO Larry Fink Says He Believes in 'Forcing Behaviors,'" YouTube, March 31, 2022, https://www.youtube.com/wa tch?v=1mfElnS0EOg.

3. Guardian News, "'Face Masks Are Our Best Defence,' Says CDC Director Redfield," YouTube, September 16, 2020, https://www.youtube.com/ watch?v=vOClXAg9nQU; Joseph Guzman, "CDC Director Says US Can Get Coronavirus 'Under Control' in 1–2 Months If Everyone Wears Masks," *The Hill*, July 14, 2020, https://thehill.com/changing-america/well-being/prevention-cures/507344-cdc-director-says-us-can-get-coronavirus-under/.

4. John T. Brooks et al., "Maximizing Fit for Cloth and Medical Procedure Masks to Improve Performance and Reduce SARS-CoV-2 Transmission and Exposure, 2021," Centers for Disease Control and Prevention, February 19, 2021, https://www.cdc.gov/mmwr/volumes/70/wr/mm70 07e1.htm; Watts L. Dietrich et al., "Laboratory Modeling of SARS-CoV-2 Exposure Reduction through Physically Distanced Seating in Aircraft Cabins Using Bacteriophage Aerosol—November 2020," Centers for Disease Control and Prevention, April 23, 2021, https://www .cdc.gov/mmwr/volumes/70/wr/mm7016e1.htm.

5. "Press Briefing by White House COVID-19 Response Team and Public Health Officials," The White House, December 17, 2021, https://www.whi tehouse.gov/briefing-room/press-briefings/2021/12/17/press-briefing-by -white-house-covid-19-response-team-and-public-health-officials-74/.

6. Josh Holder, "Tracking Coronavirus Vaccinations around the World," *New York Times*, June 28, 2022, https://www.nytimes.com/interactive /2021/world/covid-vaccinations-tracker.html.

Chapter 21: Lockdowns Taught Us We Are All in This Together! WRONG.

1. Eli Rapoport et al., "Reporting of Child Maltreatment during the SARS-CoV-2 Pandemic in New York City from March to May 2020," *Child Abuse & Neglect* 116, no. 104719 (2021): 1–7, https://www.sciencedirect.com/science/article/pii/S0145213420303744?via%3Dihub.

2. Ryan Prior, "1 in 4 Young People Are Reporting Suicidal Thoughts. Here's How to Help," CNN Health, August 15, 2020, https://edition.cnn.com/2020/08/14/health/young-people-suicidal-ideation-wellness/index.html; Nirmita Panchal, Robin Rudowitz, and Cynthia Cox, "Recent Trends in Mental Health and Substance Use Concerns among Adolescents," Kaiser Family Foundation, June 28, 2022, https://www.kff.org/coronavirus-covid-19/issue-brief/recent-trends-in-mental-health-and-substance-use-concerns-among-adolescents/.

3. Jonas Herby, Lars Jonung, and Steve H. Hanke, "A Literature Review and Meta-Analysis of the Effects of Lockdowns on COVID-19 Mortality," Studies in Applied Economics, No. 200, January 2022, https://sites.krieger.jhu.edu/iae/files/2022/01/A-Literature-Review-and-Meta-Analysis-of-the-Effects-of-Lockdowns-on-COVID-19-Mortality.pdf.

4. Consider these lists of lockdown impacts documented in scholarly journals or noted in various publications:

    People Suffering from Other Diseases
    1.4 million additional tuberculosis deaths due to lockdown disruptions
    500,000 additional deaths related to HIV
    Malaria deaths could double to 770,000 total per year
    65 percent decrease in all cancer screenings
    Breast cancer screenings dropped 89 percent
    Colorectal screenings dropped 85 percent
    Projected increase in cancer deaths, including up to 16.6 percent increase in colorectal cancer deaths, 9.5 percent increase in breast cancer

deaths, and 5.4 percent increase in lung cancer deaths over the next 5 years

75 percent decrease in suspected cancer referrals in the UK...

Widespread disruption of access to health care in the UK, disproportionately for poor

Increase in cardiac arrests but decrease in EMS calls for them

38% decrease in heart disease–related treatments

33% drop in heart attack patients, 58% drop in stroke patients

Significant increase in stress-related cardiomyopathy during lockdowns

By mid-October [2020], 3 million people in the UK had missed out on cancer screenings since the start of the pandemic

Starvation and Food Insecurity

168k child hunger deaths predicted in Africa

As many as 12,000 additional hunger deaths expected per day globally due to lockdown disruptions, up to 6,000 children

World Food Programme sees an 82% increase in food insecurity.

132 million additional people in sub-Saharan Africa are projected to be undernourished due to lockdown disruptions.

More than 50 million people living in America, including 17 million children, are likely to experience food insecurity by the end of the year

UNICEF is having to feed UK children for the first time

2 million Filipino families are starving because of lockdowns, at levels "never seen before"

UN warns that the famine and lockdown fallout in 2021 will be catastrophic

Effects on Children

Study estimates up to 2.3 million additional child deaths in the next year from lockdowns

Lockdowns are fueling child labor, including in commercial sex exploitation, mining, and tobacco production

Up to 104% increase in new HIV infections among children

Millions of girls have been deprived of access to food, basic healthcare, and protection, and thousands exposed to abuse and exploitation

FGM increases in Africa, setting back previous widespread efforts to end FGM

Lockdown estimate: an estimated 13 million more child marriages

Teen pregnancy up in many countries

Low-income students are suffering in online classes, widening inequality

School closures leading to a disproportionate [increase in] health, social, and economic divides between low- and high-income families

School closures in the US decreased reported child abuse by 27 percent

Billions of days of lost education worldwide

Decreased access to healthcare

Anxiety and stress from stay-at-home orders

Sharp rise in eating disorders among children

Child abuse reports increased 34% in Ireland between March and December

Children, in greater numbers and at younger ages, are facing suicide and drug problems in Bradford, UK, due to lockdowns

Domestic/Sexual Abuse

Domestic violence reports have skyrocketed

Up to 70% decrease in reports of child abuse to CPS early in lockdown

Male victim domestic abuse calls increased by 60% in the UK

Domestic abuse becomes more severe during lockdowns

Economy and Poverty

150 million people forced into extreme poverty

8 million Americans pushed into poverty—largest increase in US history

Half of lower-income Americans report household job or wage loss due to lockdowns

A year of lockdowns has destroyed a decade of progress in helping the world's poor—particularly children

Shutdowns cause disproportionate number of evictions for Black and Latino tenants

School closures are causing many detrimental second-order economic effects

Lockdowns drive homelessness in NYC to record levels

Over 110,000 US restaurants permanently closed

Unemployment tripled among young Americans, 52% now live with their parents

2 million UK families have been pushed into poverty

NYC bankruptcies are up 40% compared to a year ago (as of September)

Half of European small and medium businesses say they will face bankruptcy in the next year

New Zealand lockdowns pushed 70k children into poverty

90% of New Zealanders who lost their jobs were women

Thousands of Aucklanders turn to food banks—there are now 29 registered food banks in Auckland; prior to COVID there were less than 5

Up to 500,000 fewer births in the U.S. will create severe economic hardship for childcare and child-related services and products

The end of 2020 brought the sharpest rise in the U.S. poverty rate since the 1960s

The equivalent of 225 million full-time jobs lost in 2020 according to the UN

Lockdowns created a "lost generation of unemployed" as those over 50 lose careers

Mental health

1 in 5 U.S. adults developed mental disorder

1 in 4 young adults have seriously considered suicide

Severe consequences from isolation of the elderly—increased mortality, worsening cognitive abilities, accelerating dementia, mental health consequences, failure to thrive, etc.

Isolation of children significantly increases their risk of poor adult health—both mentally and physically

Half of young adults showing signs of depression

Half of students say their mental health has declined

Suicidal ideation increased in areas under stay-at-home orders while it remained stable in areas that did not have stay-at-home orders

Cases of depression and prevalence of depression symptoms have tripled in the U.S.

As many as 10 million people, including 1.5 million children, are thought to need new or additional mental health support as a direct result of lockdowns in the UK

70% increase in referrals of patients with serious suicidal thoughts in Israel

A survey of college students showed ~ 85% experienced high to moderate levels of distress

In New Zealand, cases of depression and anxiety rose substantively in the wake of lockdowns

In England, 44.6% of 17–22 year-olds with probable mental health problems reported not seeking help because of the pandemic

Suicides

Suicide-related calls to crisis hotline in Canada increased 66%

Suicides up in Bay Area

Projected increase in suicides in Canada

Suicides up sharply in Toronto

Canadians in quarantine twice as likely to have suicidal thoughts

Military suicides up 20%

Suicides increasing among children in Dallas metro area

Male suicides at highest level in two decades in England

Suicides rising in Japan for the first time in over a decade

Three times as many fentanyl deaths in Clark County, NV compared to 2019

Overdose deaths have spiked in San Francisco during lockdowns

Substance Abuse

Overdoses and overdose deaths are at their highest point ever for a 12-month period in the United States

Canada seeing record number of opioid deaths (Alberta, British Columbia, Winnipeg, Saskatchewan)

More people are needing drugs to cope with anxiety and depression

Fentanyl overdoses increased 60% in Georgia since lockdown

Every week of lockdowns increases binge drinking by 19%

This list is from "The Truth about Lockdowns," Rational Ground, July 6, 2021, https://rationalground.com/the-truth-about-lockdowns/.

5.   Eliza Barclay, Dylan Scott, and Christina Animashaun, "The US Doesn't Just Need to Flatten the Curve. It Needs to 'Raise the Line.,'" *Vox*, April 7, 2020, https://www.vox.com/2020/4/7/21201260/coronavirus-usa-chart-mask-shortage-ventilators-flatten-the-curve.

6.   Kieran Gallagher et al., "Early 2021 Data Show No Rebound in Health Care Utilization," Peterson-KFF Health System Tracker, August 17, 2021, https://www.healthsystemtracker.org/brief/early-2021-data-show-no-rebound-in-health-care-utilization/; Stinson Norwood (@snorman1776), "I would just like to remind you…," Twitter, June 25, 2022, 4:35 p.m., https://twitter.com/snorman1776/status/15407958126 27742721?s=20&t=28CrIpXoG5tseTD44MNcqA.

7.   Matt Malkus (@malkusm), "March 2021 FAIR Health Study: Total claims for ages 13–18 . . . ," (thread) Twitter, March 23, 2022, 6:44 p.m., https://twitter.com/malkusm/status/1506763901752553481; FAIR Health, *The Impact of COVID-19 on Pediatric Mental Health* (New York: FAIR Health, 2021), https://s3.amazonaws.com/media2.fairhealth.org/whitepaper/asset/The%20Impact%20of%20COVID-19%20on%20Pediatric%20Mental%20Health%20-%20A%20Study%20of%20Private%20Healthcare%20Claims%20-%20A%20FAIR%20Health%20White%20Paper.pdf.

Chapter 22: The Pandemic Led to Lots of Sex and a Baby Boom! WRONG.

1. Carly Severn, "Dating and Sex during Coronavirus: From Masks to Kissing, a Guide to Your Risks," KQED, July 10, 2020, https://www.kq ed.org/news/11826988/sex-and-dating-during-coronavirus-from-masks -to-kissing-a-guide-to-your-risks.

2. In Oregon the health overlords of that state put out some kindly advice for relationships in 2021. Step one of course is to get vaccinated. For step two the Oregon Health Authority ponders aloud: "If Zoom dates aren't cutting it, consider outdoor activities." They just assume that you've already gotten to first base. Or possibly farther. With, essentially, yourself. Step three: If your date has symptoms *cancel, cancel, cancel*! Step four: Mask up and keep your distance. Step five: Be careful but go ahead and have sex. If you dare. "Taking Extra Precautions while Dating during COVID-19," Oregon.gov, September 23, 2021, https://covidblog.oregon .gov/taking-extra-precautions-while-dating-during-covid-19/.

    Can you imagine this scene playing out in Peninsula Park in Portland? Between the riots and rallying cries of the BLM protests, two stricken lovebirds, clad in masks, holding their shot-sore arms, socially distanced, and yelling sweet nothings to each other: "I think it's safe if we're intimate, don't you?" says he. She answers: "Are you fourteen days past your booster shot?" They might get hit by a flying brick next, but at least they died Covid-free.

3. "Safer Sex and COVID-19," NYC Health, October 13, 2021, https:// www1.nyc.gov/assets/doh/downloads/pdf/imm/covid-sex-guidance.pdf; "COVID-19 and Sex: Tips for Staying Safe," StoryMD, https://storymd .com/journal/wxlrnl41zw/page/g25q6ksno4nz.

4. "Sex during the COVID-19 Public Health Emergency," Government of the District of Columbia, https://coronavirus.dc.gov/sex.

5. "Sexual Health during COVID-19," Austin Public Health, https://www .austintexas.gov/sites/default/files/files/Sexual%20Health%20-%20Fly er_Final.pdf.

6. "Sex and COVID-19," American Sexual Health Association, August 20, 2020, https://www.ashasexualhealth.org/sex-in-the-time-of-covid-19/.

7. Mark Steyn, *America Alone: The End of the World as We Know It* (Washington, D.C.: Regnery, 2006).

8. Justin Hart, "No Kids to Stick the Bill To," Rational Ground (Substack), October 8, 2021, https://covidreason.substack.com/p/no-kids-to-stick -the-bill-to; "'infertility': Search term," Google Trends, June 29, 2022, https://trends.google.com/trends/explore?date=today%205-y&geo=US &q=infertility.

9. For the month of February across the years 2015 to 2021 we see:

    2015: 37,377

    2016: 37,866

    2017: 36,091

    2018: 34,551

    2019: 34,019

    2020: 33,315

    Why February? Backtrack nine months from February and you end up right in the middle of the California stay-at-home orders.

    Justin Hart (@justin_hart), "California births for Feb 2015–21....," Twitter, January 17, 2022, 3:08 p.m., https://twitter.com/justin_hart/ status/1483169457354665984; "Natality Information," Centers for Disease Control and Prevention, November 24, 2021, https://wonder.cdc. gov/natality.html.

10. "'infertility': Search term"; Hart, "No Kids to Stick the Bill To."

Chapter 23: During Covid, All Lives Matter! WRONG.

1. Jennifer Nuzzo, DrPH (@JenniferNuzzo), "We should always evaluate the risks and benefits...," Twitter, June 2, 2020, 2:25 p.m., https://twi tter.com/JenniferNuzzo/status/1267885076697812993?s=20&t=CYqr NkzmWqIjcgpP3MHnnQ.

2. NBC News (@NBCNews), "Rally for Black trans lives...," Twitter, June 14, 2020, 4:50 p.m., https://twitter.com/NBCNews/status/12722

70112045834240?s=20&t=CYqrNkzmWqIjcgpP3MHnnQ; Doha Madani, "Rally for Black Trans Lives Draws Enormous Crowd in Brooklyn," June 14, 2020, https://www.nbcnews.com/feature/nbc-out/rally-black-trans-lives-draws-packed-crowd-brooklyn-museum-plaza-n1231040?cid=sm_npd_nn_tw_mahart/status/1483169457354665984; NBC News (@NBCNews), "President Trump plans to rally his supporters…," Twitter, June 14, 2020, 6:13 p.m., https://twitter.com/NBCNews/status/1272290986086014984?s=20&t=CYqrNkzmWqIjcgpP3MHnnQ.

3.   Tal Axelrod, "California Gov. Newsom Calls for Statewide Use-of-Force Standard," *The Hill*, June 5, 2020, https://thehill.com/homenews/state-watch/501428-california-gov-newsom-calls-for-statewide-use-of-force-standard/.

4.   Justin Hart (@justin_hart), "This is brilliant.…," Twitter, June 9, 2020, 11:09 a.m., https://twitter.com/justin_hart/status/1270372490758328320?s=20&t=CYqrNkzmWqIjcgpP3MHnnQ.

5.   Ibid.

Chapter 24: "Covid Karens" Really Have Everyone's Best Interest at Heart! WRONG.

1.   Here are some stories Rational Ground readers related:

"My family and I were up skiing and we were sitting on the gondola. This woman steps up and as she's loading on the gondola she loudly says 'Everyone in here is vaccinated, RIGHT?!' As the doors closed and she took her seat, I looked her in the eye and said, 'No, my son and I are not vaccinated.' The doors were already closed. She looked at me horrified. She looked at me horrified and I spent the entire ride up the mountain fake coughing. Not nice, but oh so satisfactory."

Another reader describes a confrontational encounter at a grocery store. She stood her ground: "My worst Karen encounter happened at the grocery store. We were waiting in line to checkout, not wearing masks because we knew the employees won't say anything about it. When this dude starts complaining about other people in line because they weren't wearing their mask over their noses. He's going on and on about how he has a heart condition and is immune compromised. The other customers pull up their masks. We were chuckling to ourselves because he hadn't seen us yet, totally maskless. When he finally sees us he starts yelling at us. Saying we were trying to kill him. I just yelled back that the masks were useless. Stood my ground. Mind you I'm 5-ft nothing."

One must wonder how we survived one hundred years without wearing masks. Grocery stores were seemingly ground zero for confrontations: "I was at the grocery store with mask below my nose looking at produce and minding my own business. Some man, out of the blue started yelling at me in front of others saying, 'You're the reason we're in this mess, you're the problem!' I was so shocked and mortified. I am a super harmless looking and small mom type. I guess I seemed like easy prey. Instead of reacting, I just stared him down silent until he backed away. A nearby gentleman gave me a high five for not engaging with someone clearly unhinged."

2.   Justin Hart (@justin_hart), "We've lost our ever-lovin' minds. . . . ," Twitter, December 25, 2020, 11:46 p.m., https://twitter.com/justin_hart/status/1342693346750283776?s=20&t=i0dfVx6bey1SNkfrmlFZ1Q.

3.   TNK (@TTBikeFit), "I'll close with two more Slavitt gems . . . ," Twitter, January 16, 2021, 5:51 p.m., https://twitter.com/TTBikeFit/status/1350576445291167748?s=20&t=i0dfVx6bey1SNkfrmlFZ1Q.

4.   Ibid.

5.   Curtis Houck (@CurtisHouck), "CBS segment on #Thanksgiving suggests families...," Twitter, November 24, 2021, 11:06 a.m., https://twitter.com/CurtisHouck/status/1463539499397431306?s=20&t=i0dfVx6bey1SNkfrmlFZ1Q.

Chapter 25: You Must Keep Sacrificing to Quell the Disease! WRONG.

1. Alexis de Toqueville, *Democracy in America*, trans. Henry Reeve, vol. 2 (1899; Charlottesville: University of Virginia, 1997), section 2, chapter 4, https://xroads.virginia.edu/~Hyper/DETOC/ch2_04.htm.

2. Paul Elias Alexander, "More than 400 Studies on the Failure of Compulsory Covid Interventions (Lockdowns, Restrictions, Closures)," Brownstone Institute, November 30, 2021, https://brownstone.org/arti cles/more-than-400-studies-on-the-failure-of-compulsory-covid-interv entions/.

3. "The Face Masks," *Des Moines Evening Tribune*, November 30, 1918, https://www.newspapers.com/clip/49066065/.

4. Steven Lemongello, Richard Tribou, and Ryan Gillespie, "DeSantis Suspends All Local COVID Orders, Signs Bill Handcuffing Cities, Counties on Future Restrictions," *Orlando Sentinel*, May 3, 2021, https://www.orlandosentinel.com/politics/os-ne-desantis-press-confere nce-may-3-20210503-os2hkcokavddvdoukcmqaply5q-story.html.

Chapter 26: Covid Is like Nothing We've Ever Seen Before! WRONG.

1. Dillon Thompson, "City Officials Fill Iconic Venice Beach Skate Park with Sand: 'We're Doing This for Our Safety,'" Yahoo! Life, April 20, 2020, https://www.yahoo.com/lifestyle/2020-04-20-venice-beach-ska te-park-filled-sand-los-angeles-government-24048865.html; BROTHERS MARSHALL, "(OFFICIAL VIDEO) S.U.P. PADDLE BOARDER ARRESTED FOR SURFING MALIBU," YouTube, April 4, 2020, https://www.youtube.com/watch?v=5moFsYVdHVo. Here are two of the more famous cases:

February 2021: In Lancaster, California, a state health official has just told a microbrewery that they will have to close down. As the front staff clamored to rouse the owners, video cameras captured the health inspector doing a little happy dance at the thought of her latest obtained scalp. Fox News, "Health Inspector Caught on Camera Allegedly Dancing after Shutting Down Brewery," YouTube, February 17, 2021, https://www.youtube.com/watch?v=P1Bj7J0kQqk.

September 2021: The California Department of Public Health puts out an advisory for people to put their masks back on their faces in between bites when dining out. Office of the Governor of California (@CAgovernor), "Going out to eat with members of your household…," Twitter, October 3, 2020, 1:00 p.m., https://twitter.com/CAgovernor/status/1312437371460173825?s=20&t=iodfVx6bey1SNkfrmlFZ1Q.

2. Alessandro Manzoni, *I Promessi Sposi (The Betrothed)* (New York: P. F. Collier & Son Company, 1909–14; Bartlby.com, 2001), chapter 31, https://www.bartleby.com/21/31.html.

3. Ibid., chapter 32, https://www.bartleby.com/21/32.html.

4. Personal communication with two California restaurant owners.

5. Don Thompson, "Nearly a Third of California's Restaurants Permanently Closed as Pandemic Set In," ABC7, May 19, 2021, https://abc7.com/restaurants-coronavirus-pandemic-covid/10663697/.

6. Manzoni, *I Promessi Sposi*, chapter 32.

7. Ian Miller (@ianmSC), "And I often hear that Australia's fine with cases now…," Twitter, January 17, 2022, 1:03 p.m., https://twitter.com/ianmSC/status/1483138042164432897?s=20&t=CYqrNkzmWqIjcgpP3MHnnQ.

8. Manzoni, *I Promessi Sposi*, chapter 32.

Chapter 27: The Rollout of Vaccines Was Bumpy but Fair! WRONG.

1. "COVID-19 Vaccination Program Interim Operational Guidance Jurisdiction Operations," Centers for Disease Control and Prevention, October 29, 2020, https://www.cdc.gov/vaccines/imz-managers/downloads/Covid-19-Vaccination-Program-Interim_Playbook.pdf.

2. Shannon Caturano and Alyssa Paolicelli, "Cuomo Threatens $1M Fine for Vaccine Fraud; COVID-19 Infection Rate Jumps," Spectrum News

NY1, December 29, 2020, https://www.ny1.com/nyc/all-boroughs/coro navirus/2020/12/28/cuomo-to-order--1m-for-vaccine-fraud--covid-19 -infection-rate-jumps.

3. "CDC to Reverse Course and Follow Florida's Lead Prioritizing 'Seniors First' for Vaccinations," Ron DeSantis: 46th Governor of Florida, January 12, 2021, https://www.flgov.com/2021/01/12/cdc-to-reverse-co urse-and-follow-floridas-lead-prioritizing-seniors-first-for-vaccinations/.

4. Ibid.

Chapter 28: Government Scientists Are Doing Okay, Considering the Challenge! WRONG.

1. "Disturbing Videos Claim to Show People Collapsing in Wuhan," read one headline in early 2020 from the *Daily Mail*. Chris Pleasance, "Do These Videos Show People Collapsing in the Streets of Wuhan?," *Daily Mail*, January 24, 2020, https://www.dailymail.co.uk/news/article-792 3981/Coronavirus-Disturbing-videos-claim-people-collapsing-Wuhan .html. The BBC ran a series titled *Coronavirus: A Visual Guide to the Outbreak*. Similar stories appeared throughout the world press. Even Snopes, always ready to tag a claim as false, gave these headlines the far-from-benign denotation of "Unproven." Dan Evon, "Are People Collapsing in the Street from Coronavirus?," Snopes, January 30, 2020, https://www.snopes.com/fact-check/people-collapsing-coronavirus/.

2. "Coronavirus: Residents 'Welded' inside Their Own Homes in China," LBC News, February 2, 2020, https://www.lbc.co.uk/news/coronavirus -residents-welded-inside-their-own-home/.

3. David Cyranoski, "What China's Coronavirus Response Can Teach the Rest of the World," *Nature* 579 (March 26, 2020): 479–80, https://www .nature.com/articles/d41586-020-00741-x.

4. See World Health Organization, *Report of the WHO-China Joint Mission on Coronavirus Disease 2019 (COVID-19)* (Geneva: World Health Organization, 2020), 19, https://www.who.int/docs/default-sou rce/coronaviruse/who-china-joint-mission-on-covid-19-final-report.pdf;

see also Michael P. Senger's report on a vast array of Chinese propaganda and WHO water carrying here: Michael P. Senger, "China's Global Lockdown Propaganda Campaign," Tablet, September 15, 2020, https://www.tabletmag.com/sections/news/articles/china-covid-lockdown-propaganda.

5. "Coronavirus: Satellie Traffic Images May Suggest Virus Hit Wuhan Earlier," BBC News, June 9, 2020, https://www.bbc.com/news/world-us-canada-52975934.

6. World Health Organization (WHO) (@WHO), "At this stage, there is no clear evidence…," Twitter, January 12, 2020, 11:31 a.m., https://twitter.com/WHO/status/1216397232427147264?s=20&t=VgGJpLFx2UKm_a5SBg-bgA.

7. D. T. Max, "The Chinese Workers Who Assemble Designer Bags in Tuscany," *New Yorker*, April 9, 2018, https://www.newyorker.com/magazine/2018/04/16/the-chinese-workers-who-assemble-designer-bags-in-tuscany.

8. Helen Davidson, "Senior WHO Adviser Appears to Dodge Question on Taiwan's Covid-19 Response," *The Guardian*, March 30, 2020, https://www.theguardian.com/world/2020/mar/30/senior-who-adviser-appears-to-dodge-question-on-taiwans-covid-19-response.

9. "WHO Director-General's Statement on IHR Emergency Committee on Novel Coronavirus (2019-nCoV)," World Health Organization, January 30, 2020, https://www.who.int/director-general/speeches/detail/who-director-general-s-statement-on-ihr-emergency-committee-on-novel-coronavirus-(2019-ncov).

10. Benjamin Fearnow, "Mike Pompeo Rejects 'Corrupt' WHO Findings That COVID Didn't Originate in Wuhan Lab," *Newsweek*, February 9, 2021, https://www.newsweek.com/mike-pompeo-rejects-corrupt-who-findings-that-covid-didnt-originate-wuhan-lab-1567946.

Chapter 29: The Pandemic Brings Out the Best in Our Leaders! WRONG.

1. Caitlin O'Kane, "Stars Attending VMAs in New York City Will Not Have to Quarantine like Others Traveling from COVID-19 Hot Spots," CBS News, August 24, 2020, https://www.cbsnews.com/news/mtv-vid eo-music-awards-new-york-city-no-quarantine/.

2. Brooke Singman, "Pelosi Used Shuttered San Francisco Hair Salon for Blow-Out, Owner Calls It 'Slap in the Face,'" Fox News, September 2, 2020, https://www.foxnews.com/politics/pelosi-san-francisco-hair-sal on-owner-calls-it-slap-in-the-face.

3. Bill Melugin and Shelly Insheiwat, "FOX 11 Obtains Exclusive Photos of Gov. Newsom at French Restaurant Allegedly Not Following COVID-19 Protocols," FOX 11 Los Angeles, November 17, 2020, https://www .foxla.com/news/fox-11-obtains-exclusive-photos-of-gov-newsom-at-fr ench-restaurant-allegedly-not-following-covid-19-protocols.

4. Examples include:

    In San Francisco, it was revealed that city government employees could enjoy the privilege of office building gyms while private gyms were forced to shut their doors. Trisha Thadani, "SFPD Gyms Have Remained Open during the Pandemic. So Why Are Private Ones Still Closed?," *San Francisco Chronicle*, September 4, 2020, https://www.sfchronicle.com /politics/article/SFPD-gyms-have-remained-open-during-the-pandemic -15542002.php.

    In Alexandria City, Virginia, the superintendent of schools put his daughter in a private school so that she might have access to in-person learning, something he prevented the public schools he oversaw from doing. Nikki Harris, "Exclusive: ACPS Superintendent Hutchings Sends Child To Private School Bishop Ireton," *Theogony*, October 7, 2020, https://www.acpsk12.org/theogony/2020-2021/2020/10/07/exclusive-ac ps-superintendent-hutchings-sends-child-to-private-school-bishop-ireton/.

    Like many members of Congress, private travel keeps you away from the rabble. In September 2020, California senator Diane Feinstein was seen entering a private airplane terminal without wearing a mask. Her staff, the crew, and the pilots were all fully masked, of course. Evie Fordham and Alex Pfeiffer, "Feinstein Spotted without Mask at Dulles Airport despite Calls for 'Mandatory' Policy," Fox News, September 29, 2020, https://www.foxnews.com/politics/dianne-feinstein-no-mask-tucker-carlson.

In El Paso, Texas, a city attorney said that citizens need to take responsibility to stop the COVID-19 crisis. She was then outed on social media hosting a maskless birthday party with her daughter with members of outside families—a big no-no under those city's guidelines. Keenan Willard, "City Officials Defend Alleged Gathering Hosted by El Paso City Attorney," KFOX14, November 12, 2020, https://kfoxtv.com/news/coronavirus/city-officials-defend-alleged-gathering-hosted-by-el-paso-city-attorney.

Lori Lightfoot, who never met a lockdown policy she didn't like, defended a street party she held as a rally for Joe Biden, infringing several of her own lockdown policies. Douglas Ernst, "Lori Lightfoot Denies Virus Hypocrisy of Attending Pro-Biden Street Party; Crowd Needed 'Relief,'" *Washington Times*, November 13, 2020, https://www.washingtontimes.com/news/2020/nov/13/lori-lightfoot-denies-virus-hypocrisy-of-attending/.

Governor Andrew Cuomo, who would resign in disgrace, first solidified his stature as hypocrite-in-chief by planning to host his eighty-nine-year-old grandma for Thanksgiving—something he forbade other New Yorkers from doing. He would later admit that he traveled to Mississippi where his own daughters had fled—something, again, that he strongly encouraged New Yorkers NOT to do. Kaylee McGhee White, "Here's a List of All the Democratic Officials Who Have Defied Their Own Coronavirus Restrictions," *Washington Examiner*, December 1, 2020, https://www.washingtonexaminer.com/opinion/heres-a-list-of-all-the-democratic-officials-who-have-defied-their-own-coronavirus-restrictions.

In November 2020, the mayor of Denver, Michael B. Hancock, was seen waiting for a plane at Denver International Airport. His official account tweeted out at that same hour: "Avoid travel, if you can." Andrea Salcedo, "Denver's Mayor Urged Residents to Avoid Thanksgiving Travel. Then He Flew Cross-Country to See Family," *Washington Post*, November 26, 2020, https://www.washingtonpost.com/nation/2020/11 /26/denver-mayor-hancock-thanksgiving-covid/.

That same month, Los Angeles supervisor Sheila Kuehl voted to ban all outdoor dining, something she described as "a most dangerous situation." Hours before the vote, she was seen dining at *Il Forno Trattoria* in Santa Monica. She later excused herself saying that she wanted to be one of the first ones to tell the restaurant staff the bad news. Bill Melugin, "LA County Supervisor Dines at Restaurant Hours after Voting to Ban Outdoor Dining," FOX11 Los Angeles, November 30, 2020, https:// www.foxla.com/news/la-county-supervisor-dines-at-restaurant-hours-af ter-voting-to-ban-outdoor-dining.

The mayor of Austin, Texas, Steve Adler told the public in a Facebook video to "stay home if you can…this is not the time to relax." He did not disclose that the video was made on vacation in Cabo San Lucas. Tony Plohetski (@tplohetski), "EXCLUSIVE: Austin Mayor Steve Adler told the public…," Twitter, December 2, 2020, 2:40 p.m., https://twitter.com /tplohetski/status/1334221005607362568?s=20&t=VgGJpLFx2UKm _a5SBg-bgA.

Dr. Deborah Birx, the key advisor on the Covid-19 taskforce, warned Americans about traveling over Thanksgiving. It was later revealed that she traveled and met three generations of her family at her own Thanksgiving celebration. Aamer Madhani and Brian Slodysko, "Birx Travels, Family Visits Highlight Pandemic Safety Perils," AP News, December 20, 2020, https://apnews.com/article/travel-pandemics-only -on-ap-delaware-thanksgiving-52810c22488fff7e6bb70746bdc9bc61.

Sarah Chambers, an executive who sits on the board of the Chicago Teacher's Union, snapped a fun selfie on a beach while not in Chicago after strongly encouraging all teachers to stay home and stay safe. Corey A. DeAngelis (@DeAngelisCorey), "'Sarah Chambers is on the union's executive board…,'" Twitter, January 1, 2021, 11:22 a.m., https://twitter.com/DeAngelisCorey/status/1345042738828476416?s=20&t=VgGJpLFx2UKm_a5SBg-bgA.

In the UK news reports was found the fine print of stay-at-home orders that allowed for senior executives of various companies to leave quarantine if the activities had "significant financial benefit." "Importers and Exporters: Financial Sanctions—Frequently Asked Questions," Gov.UK, December 13, 2021, https://www.gov.uk/government/publications/ofsi-guidance-html-documents/importers-and-exporters-financial-sanctions-frequently-asked-questions; Beth Timmins, "Smaller Firms Express Anger at Quarantine Exemption Plans for Big Business," BBC News, June 29, 2021, https://www.bbc.com/news/business-57644437.

Texas Democratic lawmakers employed a tactic to stall a bill in the local legislature by leaving the state altogether. They traveled on a private plane and took selfies, maskless of course. Alex Ura and Cassandra Pollock, "Texas House Democrats Flee the State in Move That Could Block Voting Restrictions Bill, Bring Legislature to a Halt," The Texas Tribune, July 12, 2021, https://www.texastribune.org/2021/07/12/texas-democrats-voting-bill-quorum/.

In August 2021 numerous celebrities and lawmakers were seen at former president Obama's birthday bash—all of them maskless. Hannah Yasharoff, "Barack Obama Celebrates at 60th Birthday Bash after Scaling Back Guest List Because of Covid Concerns," *USA Today*, August 8, 2021, https://www.usatoday.com/story/entertainment/celebrities/2021/08/08/barack-obama-birthday-former-president-celebrates-60-amid-covid-rise/5530559001/.

London Breed, the mayor of San Francisco, presided over perhaps the most stringent Covid policies any city had witnessed in the United States. She was caught on camera numerous times, maskless and cavorting inside against her own policies. Robby Soave, "More COVID-19 Hypocrisy:

San Francisco Mayor London Breed Partied Maskless at a Jazz Club," *Reason*, September 17, 2021, https://reason.com/2021/09/17/london-br eed-san-francisco-mask-covid-hypocrisy/.

5.   "WEAR YOUR MASK! COMMANDS DRASTIC NEW ORDINANCE," (headline) *San Francisco Chronicle*, October 25, 1918, https://www.newspapers.com/clip/47294075/san-francisco-chronicle/.

6.   The headline in the *Santa Barbara Daily News and the Independent* on November 16, 1918, was "MASK IS CHIEF ALLY OF 'FLU' PHYSICIANS DECLARE." The teaser before the article reads, "Average Person Doesn't Know How to Take Care of Mask and It Becomes Veritable Bacteria Incubator." https://www.newspapers.com/clip/10050 9906/mask-if-chief-ally-of-flu-physicians/.

Let's hop over to Iowa and the *Des Moines Tribune* of November 30, 1918. A writer submitted a poem called "The Song of the Mask":

Smile at me only with thine eyes,

Dear heart, they've put the mask

On lips that often tantalize,

All who in your smiles bask.

Those teeth of pearl are hid from view;

That dimpled chin we miss;

And all because the blasted flu

Has brought the town to this.

So smile, dear heart, with twinkling eyes;

No law can cover those;

They lift my hopes unto the skies

And keep me on my toes.

The days will pass, the flu will go,

And masks will drop once more;

We'll smile and laugh again, and so

Forget that we were sore.

Furthermore, mask jokes were all the rage. From that same issue of the *Des Moines Tribune*: "One badgered benedict wants to know why they don't extend the wearing of the flu masks to the home so he won't know whether his wife greets him with a smile or a frown when he arrives late for dinner."

The jokes continue: "It wouldn't be difficult now to organize a local branch of the Ku-Klux-Klan in Des Moines," and "Those girls who lament constantly the absence of a 'decisive' chin might try wearing flu masks with special chin pads. (Patent applied for.)"

And "Maidens with masks keep a man wildly guessing, wondering if facial beauty he's missing. With lips made alone for ecstatic kissing."

Des Moines Evening Tribune, November 30, 1918, https://www.new spapers.com/clip/104698029/.

Shades of Team Apocalypse here: "Sir: Would you say that folks unduly excited over the present epidemic act like a lot of flunatics?"

7.   "Laughed at Idea," *San Francisco Chronicle*, October 25, 1918, https:// www.newspapers.com/clip/104698216/san-francisco-chronicle/.

8.   In 1919 the mayor of Oakland was arrested and fined five dollars for not properly wearing his influenza mask against city mandates he supported. Erika Mailman, "In 1919, the Mayor of Oakland Was Arrested for Failing to Wear a Mask," *Smithsonian*, May 21, 2020, https://www.smithsonianmag.com/ history/when-mayor-oakland-was-arrested-failing-wear-mask-180974950/.

In San Francisco much discussion was had over potential shutdowns and whether locales should hold school or even shut down school altogether. Principals offered the teaching staff of each school to answer urgent calls in the neighborhood. Plans were also made for the use of the kitchens of the domestic science departments in the various schools to provide food for the sick.

"Some objection was voiced at the outset to the idea of an indoor meet- ins of the teachers, but Miss Regan spoke briefly to those in the hall who were advocating the outer court as meeting place, and all went in inside."

Miss Regan is quoted as saying: "A shock is good for the nerves.... There is too much fear in San Francisco today, and too much of the idea that influenza means death. Certainly the teachers are the ones to help to a more reasonable frame of mind."

"City Teachers Volunteer Aid for Red Cross," *San Francisco Chronicle,* October 25, 1918, https://www.newspapers.com/clip/104698216/san-francisco-chronicle/.

Would that all teachers today had as much sense and bravery as this one. Unfortunately, most of our teachers' unions in this day and age continue to advocate for closed schools if cases rise.

9.   W. A. Evans, "Face Masks and Contagion: How to Keep Well," *The Spokesman-Review,* February 11, 1920, https://www.newspapers.com/clip/104698392/the-spokesman-review/.

Here's another take from *The News Journal,* Wilmington, Delaware, February 14, 1920. It's a poem, satirical in style, decrying the plethora of masks in 1920. It is titled "Masks, Masks, Who Will Buy..."

Masks! Masks!
Who will buy?
Here are masks in profusion,
All sorts and all colors, try
'Em on before a conclusion.
This one, sir? We call him Tartuffe
Why, I don't know, but the name suits;
He was a poet you think? Like enough.
We traders in masks are but brutes,
We talk prose and the jingle we love
Is a clink, money clink.
Shelley's? I think
Too removed from the fashion, a link
Betwixt hero and sainthood. Off he goes
But you choose it.
All men are fools and they show it
Under their masks!

10. "Retain Your Head Covering," *Cheraw Chronicle*, February 23, 1922, https://www.newspapers.com/clip/104698496/cheraw-chronicle/.

11. Justin Hart, "The Darkest Health Propaganda Posters," Rational Ground (Substack), October 11, 2021, https://covidreason.substack.com /p/the-darkest-health-propaganda-posters. One poster depicts the severed sleeping head of a blond woman surrounded by dreams of vegetables and fruits in a colorful splash of art with beaming sun rays lifting the entire visual. It reads: "FIGHT TURBERCULOSIS. OBEY THE RULES OF HEALTH" ("Obey" is put in the largest font to convey the urgency of this command).

Another poster depicts a stylized worker whose back is turned to us. His hand is lifted upwards as he has just tossed a pair of dice. "DON'T GAMBLE with SYPHILIS," reads the header. "CONSULT HEALTH AUTHORITIES." It's clear this fellow is going to roll snake eyes both in reality and with his chances of spreading disease.

Still another poster conveys a bit of a tattle-tale motif. A small caricature of a girls stands before a grocery counter. A man in a white behind the counter (the storekeeper) is putting apples in a bag for her. The poster admonishes: "This is the STOREKEEPER. He sells the things that are good for you to eat. He must keep the food clean." The inference here is you better keep an eye on him.

One hugely impactful moment of the Covid pandemic centered around the CDC's assertion that lack of housing was a endangerment to public health. They promptly issued an eviction moratorium that dramatically impacted the lives of millions of renters. This was a massive overreach that would eventually be struck down by the Supreme Court after having stood for over a year.

This "housing-is-health" assertion was nothing new for our government. One poster from the 1930s era depicted the figure of Death, clad in black, scythe in hand, watermarked into the back of the poster and looming over a set of brownstone public housing units. A blueprint of "Better Housing" is rolling across the poster to paper over the words: "The Solution to INFANT MORTALITY in the slums."

With a COVID-19 vaccine deep in our trenches, the continued use of masks, and the overwhelming sense that we must all find refuge bowing to social justice warriors—be warned that this type of propaganda will be making a comeback.

12. City of Santa Monica (@santamonicacity), "If you're out and about and notice a business…," Twitter, November 4, 2021, 6:00 p.m., https://twitter.com/santamonicacity/status/1456380831765835777.

Chapter 30: Government Action Saved the Economy! WRONG.

1. When it comes to toilet paper, after talking to a few people in the know, I came to realize the obvious: people do half of their "business" at their businesses. The distribution of toilet paper for commercial developments involves industrial production of the paper we've come to love. Not necessarily your soothing bear-mascot quality, but rather efficient, large quantities packaged into large reams that janitorial staff then mount in stalls in massive dispensers or efficient gizmos holding multiple rolls.

Now imagine you're an executive down at the fictitious TP supplier "Wipe World." The call comes in for the shutdown, and you have some serious decisions to make. Production managers at the Big Roll Mill (your supplier for industrial reams of TP) have shut down and will eventually furlough most of the staff. Your shipping contracts will go into default; trucks with slabs of TP rolls tightly wrapped and ready to be dispensed will be called back or even mothballed. The proverbial target of your product is about to hit the fan.

On the plus side, it turns out that profits on the consumer side of Wipe World are going to be just fine as demand outstrips supply. You stand to make a good profit if you can shift manufacturing to meet the new demand.

The marketing team is way ahead of you and pitching a product called "Wipe Forever," which comes with a freestanding mount promising you an entire month's supply of TP in one massive roll. Essentially, you repackage the industrial stock to make it consumer-friendly. (Google "Charmin Forever" if you think I'm kidding.) Problems solved—for now!

The TP shortages went on for months and would come back again and again throughout the next two years.

But the impact to the world's plumbing doesn't stop there. Michael Hurtado has spent most of his time during the pandemic flushing toilets and running water at the large Ahern property off the Vegas Strip. The fear was that as rooms stood empty, the water in the toilets and sinks would form bacteria and spread another set of nasty bugs when reopened. Elizabeth Wise, "This Man Spent Last Year Flushing Hundreds of Toilets," *USA Today*, June 23, 2021, https://www.usatoday.com/story/news/health/2021/06/08/legionnaires-disease-worry-buildings-reopen-after-covid-shutdown/5200 704001/?gnt-cfr=1.

The same scene played out across every business building, theme park, and college dorm. Engineers and janitors (the essential workers) spent their days tending the loos, minding the sinks and showers on every floor in every building. They did this not only to avoid the impact of stagnated water but to keep the plumbing going at all. Every hotel, park, skyscraper, and business office is designed with an anticipated amount of water flowing throughout the infrastructure. If and when that water stops, it can cause serious damage to an entire city's waterworks.

What's more, those pipes and sewage heroes had to deal with another blow from the domestic side of the equation. In some municipal locales clogs were up 50 percent as germ-worried households (aka, all of us in March 2020) amped up their cleaning habits and occasionally flushed those ever-present hand wipes down the john. This practice doesn't end well.

So a national shutdown leads to a run on toilet paper, caused by a sudden drop in at-work wiping, leading to massive manufacturing rework, supply-chain shifts, and a janitorial staff forced to walk the halls of vacated buildings like Jack Torrance in *The Shining,* simulating a proxy population doing their business to keep everything from falling apart. *All work and no flushing makes Michael Hurtado a very dull boy.*

2. A cycle shop owner told me, "One of my companies fits and customizes high-end bikes for competition or serious training. While low-end rec bikes sold out quickly in 2020 due to locked-down folks looking for anything to do, high-end stuff lasted a little longer and then completely disappeared. As did almost all componentry…. Some of the same brands are selling what they have direct to consumers, bypassing the bike shop networks they have relied on for decades. Shops are collapsing."

   Of course, some industries came out ahead, perhaps unexpectedly. Speaking with an electrical engineer, I found that a surprising shift in demand brought about a new type of chaos. "We spent the initial two weeks after the shutdown worrying about what we would do with construction projects," he said. "Then big corporate data center clients began realizing the lockdowns were only ramping up their business. The switch to remote work and more online ordering meant even more data center work. A nationwide home improvement client also discovered that white-collar workers stuck at home meant many people finally renovating their ugly kitchens and bathrooms; and then the housing market took off, leading to more renovations."

   Another employee of an education publisher admitted to me, "The lockdown was actually good for my work and income. I write courseware for college textbooks, and the sales went up hugely after colleges went virtual. Before 2020, courseware was an optional sales gimmick. After 2020, courseware became a crucial way of learning and grading."

3. One mother told me, "In March 2020, I was fourteen weeks pregnant with my second child, and I remember going to the grocery store for a couple items to get us through the weekend. I was met with what is best described as a run on the grocery store. So many empty shelves, so many people commenting they thought we wouldn't have food or be able to

get supplies for the next several weeks. I went in for maybe five items total and ended up with $200 of pantry staples. When I got home, I really cried for twenty minutes, and it was the lowest point of the pandemic for me. Possibly the lowest point of the pandemic for my husband, who had to watch me cry."

4. One mother said, "My son's daycare shut down ten days later and he was home for fifteen weeks while my husband and I were both working full-time. I cried several times in those subsequent weeks, mostly because I was frustrated I couldn't go out and was left at home with a needy toddler all the time."

5. Olivia Rockeman, "More than Half of U.S. Business Closures Permanent, Yelp Says," Bloomberg, July 22, 2020, https://www.bloomberg.com/news/articles/2020-07-22/more-than-half-of-u-s-business-closures-permanent-yelp-says#xj4y7vzkg. Here are some of the large companies and brand names that suffered massive failures:

    24 Hour Fitness closed over 100 gyms.

    Hertz filed bankruptcy.

    Brooks Brothers bankrupt after 200 years of service.

    California Pizza Kitchen bankrupt.

    Chuck E. Cheese bankrupt.

    Cirque du Soleil laid off nearly 400 workers.

    Dean & DeLuca downsized.

    Frontier Communications bankrupt.

    A dozen airlines bankrupt.

    GNC closed 1,200 stores.

    Gold's Gym closed 700 locations.

    J. C. Penney bankrupt, with over $4 billion in debt.

    Neiman Marcus filed for bankruptcy.

    J. Crew went bankrupt.

    So did Whiting Petroleum.

6. Madeleine Ngo, "Small Businesses Are Dying by the Thousands—and No One Is Tracking the Carnage," Bloomberg, August 11, 2020, https://www.

bloomberg.com/news/articles/2020-08-11/small-firms-die-quietly-leaving-thousands-of-failures-uncounted#xj4y7vzkg.

7. Richard Fry and Amanda Barroso, "Amid Coronavirus Outbreak, Nearly 3 in 10 Young People Are 'Disconnected,'" National Conference of State Legislatures, August 6, 2020, https://www.ncsl.org/bookstore /state-legislatures-magazine/covid-19-nearly-3-in-10-young-people-are -disconnected-magazine2020.aspx.

8. Jen Carlson, "Everything You Need to Know about Phase 3 of Reopening NYC," Gothamist, July 6, 2020, https://gothamist.com/news/everythi ng-you-need-know-about-phase-3-reopening-nyc.

9. Alex Tavlian, "Sour Grapes Emerge as Most Calif. Wineries Close while Newsom's Winery Remains Open," The San Joaquin Valley Sun, July 2, 2020, https://sjvsun.com/california/sour-grapes-emerge-as-most-calif-wineries-close-while-newsoms-winery-remains-open/.

Chapter 31: The Worst Is Over and Things Are Returning to Normal! WRONG.

1. Associated Press and Reuters, "Shanghai Residents Clash with Police over Covid-19 Measures," *New York Times*, April 15, 2022, https:// www.nytimes.com/video/world/asia/100000008306195/shanghai-china-covid-protest.html.

2. Aaron Ginn (@aginnt), "Remember they said, just two weeks….," Twitter, April 14, 2022, 10:27 p.m., https://twitter.com/aginnt/status/15 14792553039556612?s=20&t=C_-J6MN7swSv4NDJhNsang; Aaron Ginn (@aginnt), "Videos," Twitter, https://twitter.com/search?q=from %3Aaginnt%20china&src=typed_query&f=video.

3. Terrence Daniels (Captain Planet) (@Terrence_STR), "#CoronaVirus: Another Leaked Video of Chinese authorities WELDING SHUT whole apartment buildings…," Twitter, February 8, 2020, 10:48 a.m., https:// twitter.com/Terrence_STR/status/1226170838027849729?s=20&t=C_-J6MN7swSv4NDJhNsang; Things China Doesn't Want You To Know (@TruthAbtChina), "The Chinese Communist Party is welding

apartments shut…," Twitter, May 17, 2021, 5:07 p.m., https://twitter.com/TruthAbtChina/status/1394399304819757056?s=20&t=C_-J6MN7swSv4NDJhNsang; BertelSchmitt™ (@BertelSchmitt), "COVID: They are welding doors shut again in China…," Twitter, March 30, 2022, 9:33 a.m., https://twitter.com/BertelSchmitt/status/15091619213 91788032?s=20&t=C_-J6MN7swSv4NDJhNsang.

4. Scott W. Atlas, *A Plague Upon Our House: My Fight at the Trump White House to Stop COVID from Destroying America* (New York: Simon and Schuster, 2021), 291.

5. Dr. Terry McDouglas (@drterrymcd), "An idea I've has is adding a reporting function…," Twitter, September 22, 2021, 6:58 p.m., https://twitter.com/drterrymcd/status/1440812750754619397?s=20&t=8J1N sQe2MU5lxzd6XnUxXA.

6. Charlie De Mar (@CharlieDeMar), "The Hilton Chicago/Northbrook hosted a massive…," Twitter, December 2, 2020, 10:07 p.m., https://twitter.com/CharlieDeMar/status/1334333485901885440?s=20&t=8J1N sQe2MU5lxzd6XnUxXA.

7. "S6 No Lockdowns Anymore w/ Ariana Grande & Marissa Jaret Winokur," *The Late Late Show with James Corden*, CBS, June 15, 2021, https://www.cbs.com/shows/video/_RYq_E1Y3m5GHEKwCi3x _0_O27mUPvTC/.

8. "CDC Greenlights 'Mix-And-Match' Covid Boosters," Fox News, October 24, 2021, https://video.foxnews.com/v/6278601661001#sp=sh ow-clips.

9. Tom Kertscher, "In Context: 'Never Going to Learn How Safe This Vaccine Is Unless We Start Giving It,'" PolitiFact, November 1, 2021, https://www.politifact.com/article/2021/nov/01/context-never-going-le arn-how-safe-vaccine-unless-/.

10. Don Thompson, "It's a Secret: California Keeps Key Virus Data from Public," ABC News, January 22, 2021, https://abcnews.go.com/Techn ology/wireStory/secret-california-key-virus-data-public-75432129.

11. Leana Wen (@DrLeanaWen), "Joining @wolfblitzer @CNNSitRoom: Increasing vaccinations is hard…," Twitter, July 6, 2021, 6:27 p.m., https://twitter.com/drleanawen/status/1412538637418434562.

12. Caleb Hull (@CalebJHull), "Jen Psaki: We Will Be Going Door-to-Door to Americans Who Have Not Been Vaccinated," Twitter, July 6, 2021, 1:16 p.m., https://twitter.com/calebjhull/status/1412460388994670592.

13. Dr. Ellie Murray (@EpiEllie), "Trolls like to call me authoritarian for my COVID takes…," Twitter, January 14, 2022, 8:38 a.m., https://twitter.com/epiellie/status/1481984183589388299.

14. Fannie Bussieres McNicoll and Romain Schue, "Ottawa Will Ban All Unvaccinated People from Leaving Canada," Radio Canada, October 8, 2021, https://ici.radio-canada.ca/nouvelle/1830094/avion-trudeau-covid-canada-interdiction-voyage.

15. Ezra Levant (@ezralevant), "'Ottawa will prohibit all unvaccinated people from leaving Canada.' Even foreign citizens…," Twitter, October 8, 2021, 2:50 p.m., https://twitter.com/ezralevant/status/1446548564872663040.

16. "Freedom Convoy Protestors Face Suspended Insurance, Frozen Accounts under Emergencies Act," Road Today, February 16, 2022, https://www.trucknews.com/road-today/freedom-convoy-protesters-face-suspended-insurance-frozen-accounts-under-emergencies-act/.

17. Vivek Murthy (@Surgeon_General), "To create a healthier digital environment and safer future, tech companies must share what they know…," Twitter, March 7, 2022, 3:55 p.m., https://twitter.com/surgeon_general/status/1500938298306539520?lang=en.

18. "Rights Groups Petition Israel's Top Court over Omicron Phone Tracking," Reuters, November 29, 2021, https://www.reuters.com/world/middle-east/rights-groups-petition-israels-top-court-over-omicron-phone-tracking-2021-11-29/.

19. Dr. Morcease Beasley (@MorceaseBeasley), "We absolutely support the school district's decision to require masks of all even as we have rules…,"

Twitter, February 16, 2022, 6:20 p.m., https://twitter.com/MorceaseBe asley/status/1494089311884656643.

Chapter 32: What's Next

1. Conn Carroll, "We Found the Science behind Democrats' COVID Flip-Flop," *Washington Examiner*, February 25, 2022, https://www.washin gtonexaminer.com/opinion/we-found-the-science-behind-democrats-co vid-flip-flop; Julie Hamill (@hamill_law), "Here is the literal memo...," Twitter, February 25, 2022, 8:41 a.m., https://twitter.com/hamill_law/ status/1497205184790872065.

2. Jeremy Faust MD MS (ER physician) (@jeremyfaust), "The odd thing about my being disappointed...," Twitter, April 18, 2022, 7:13 p.m., https://twitter.com/jeremyfaust/status/1516193198204329984.

3. Paul Bauer (@realpaulbauer), "I'm on a southwest flight back to Sacramento and it was just announced...," Twitter, April 18, 2022, 7:56 p.m., https://twitter.com/realpaulbauer/status/1516204151629307910.

4. Barbara Morse, "Dr. Ashish Jha: 'The Pandemic Is Not Over,'" NBC 10 News WJAR, April 13, 2022, https://turnto10.com/features/health-landing-page/dr-ashish-jha-the-pandemic-is-not-over.

5. Justin Hart (@justin_hart), "Here's how it went down...," Twitter, April 18, 2022, 7:14 p.m., https://twitter.com/justin_hart/status/1516193385 706508291?s=20&t=9v4EeiLs8d2iITvNqu76SQ.

6. Bob Wachter (@Bob_Wachter), "Biden administration needs to fight this decision, even if is was gearing up to make...," Twitter, April 18, 2022, 7:55 p.m., https://twitter.com/bob_wachter/status/151620375213430 3745.

7. Jared Rabel (@JradRabel), "I boarded a plane today with my son and mid flight, the pilot announced that the mask mandate...," Twitter, April 18, 2022, 8:12 p.m., https://twitter.com/jradrabel/status/15162080129 76918537.

8. Karl Salzmann, "'This Is Maga Airspace': *New York Times* Reporter Falls Headfirst for Obvious Satire," Washington Free Beacon, April 19,

2022, https://freebeacon.com/media/this-is-maga-airspace-new-york-times-reporter-falls-headfirst-for-obvious-satire/; Jared Rabel (@JradRabel), "Just got messaged by a NYT journalist…," Twitter, April 18, 2022, 11:41 p.m., https://twitter.com/JradRabel/status/151 62605691243233333?ref_src=twsrc%5Etfw%7Ctwcamp%5Etweetemb ed%7Ctwterm%5E1516260569124323333%7Ctwgr%5E%7Ctwcon% 5Es1_&ref_url=https%3A%2F%2Ffreebeacon.com%2Fmedia%2Fthis -is-maga-airspace-new-york-times-reporter-falls-headfirst-for-obvious-satire%2F.

9.   Todd Jaquith, "NYT Journo Appears Completely Duped by Hilarious and Satirical 'This Is MAGA Airspace' Tweet," BizPacReview, April 19, 2022, https://www.bizpacreview.com/2022/04/19/nyt-journo-appears-completely-duped-by-hilarious-and-satirical-this-is-maga-airspace-tweet-1227523/.

Conclusion

1.   John P. A. Ioannidis, "A Fiasco in the Making? As the Coronavirus Pandemic Takes Hold, We Are Making Decisions without Reliable Data," Stat News, March 17, 2020, https://www.statnews.com/2020 /03/17/a-fiasco-in-the-making-as-the-coronavirus-pandemic-takes-hold -we-are-making-decisions-without-reliable-data/.

Appendix 1: Resources to Reclaim Our Ever-Loving Minds

1.   White House COVID-19 Team, Data Strategy and Execution Workgroup. 2021. *COVID-19 Community Profile Report.* Centers for Disease Control and Prevention (note included in original letter).

2.   Justin Hart, "A Letter to the Mayor of Boston, Michelle Wu," Rational Ground (Substack), December 23, 2021, https://covidreason.substack .com/p/a-letter-to-the-mayor-of-boston-michelle?s=w#_ftn1.

Appendix 2: Stories from the Pandemic

1. Michael Simonson, "People Are Literally Dying to Avoid Contracting the Coronavirus," Rational Ground, September 23, 2021, https://ration alground.com/people-are-literally-dying-to-avoid-contracting-the-coro navirus/.

2. Alex Lieske, "I'm Immunocompromised, and I've Never Asked Others to Protect Me," Rational Ground, September 19, 2021, https://rational ground.com/im-immunocompromised-and-ive-never-asked-others-to -protect-me/.

INDEX

A

administration, 18, 22, 144
 Biden, 114, 151, 159
 Trump, xii, 22, 135
agencies, 135, 153, 159, 176
 government, 40, 104, 111
Alaska, 82
Alaska Airlines, 157–58
Amazon, 144
America, United States of, 39, 57,
 95, 101, 111, 119, 163, 170,
 172
American Hospital Association,
 40
asymptomatic spread, 3, 30
Atlas, Scott, xii, 16–17, 25, 149,
 167, 209
Auchincloss, Hugh, 27–28
Australia, 56, 128
Aylward, Bruce, 135

B

baby boomers, xi, 34
Berenson, Alex, 99
Biden, Joseph, xiii, 209
Birx, Deborah, 21–22, 25–26, 61
Black Lives Matter (BLM),
 114–16
blue states, 151, 155

Breed, London, 138
bureaucrats, 5, 161
 health, 125
 unelected, xiv, 18, 163
businesses, ix, 4–7, 20, 40, 57–59,
 122, 127, 137, 140, 142–45,
 149, 152, 173, 192, 196
butterfly effect, 3

C

Canada, 151–52
cancer, 106, 183, 185, 190, 200,
 205
care pods, 79
CARES Act, 38–39
CBS, 15, 118, 149
CCP (Chinese Communist Party),
 21, 148
Centers for Disease Control and
 Prevention (CDC), 4, 7, 17, 22,
 29, 38, 41–44, 50, 57–58,
 64–66, 74–75, 94, 100, 114,
 131–32, 150, 157, 160–61, 178
Chicago, 79, 149
China, 9, 35, 133–36, 147–48,
 151, 153, 185, 192
church, xi, 126
Cigna Corporation, 205